HAND SPLINTING

Principles and methods

HAND SPLINTING
Principles and methods

ELAINE EWING FESS, M.S., O.T.R.

Hand Therapist, Consultant in Private Practice;
Founder and First Director, Hand Rehabilitation
Center of Indiana, Inc., Indianapolis, Indiana

KARAN S. GETTLE, O.T.R.

Hand Therapist and Former Director, Hand Rehabilitation
Center of Indiana, Inc., Indianapolis, Indiana

JAMES W. STRICKLAND, M.D.

Associate Professor of Orthopaedic Surgery and Director of the
Hand Surgery Rotation, Department of Orthopaedic Surgery,
Indiana University Medical School; Chief, Section of Hand Surgery,
Department of Orthopaedic Surgery, St. Vincent Hospital,
Indianapolis, Indiana

with 510 illustrations

Drawings by **Craig Gosling** and **Carol Stahl**

The C. V. Mosby Company

ST. LOUIS • TORONTO • LONDON   1981

The C. V. Mosby Company
11830 Westline Industrial Drive, St. Louis, Missouri 63146

Library of Congress Cataloging in Publication Data

Fess, Elaine Ewing, 1944-
    Hand splinting.

    Bibliography: p.
    Includes index.
    1. Hand—Surgery. 2. Splints (Surgery).
I. Gettle, Karan S., 1949-   joint author.
II. Strickland, James W., 1936-   joint author.
III. Title. [DNLM: 1. Hand injuries—Therapy.
2. Splints. WE830 P413h]
RD559. F47   617'.575'059   80-17398
ISBN 0-8016-1569-0

C/MV/MV 9 8 7 6 5 4   02/A/274

The authors dedicate this book to **Kay Bradley Carl,** OTR, whose ingenious and creative efforts resulted in the original splint manual used in the Occupational Therapy Program, Division of Allied Health Sciences, Indiana University School of Medicine. It is from this manual that this book takes its philosophic and structural orientation.

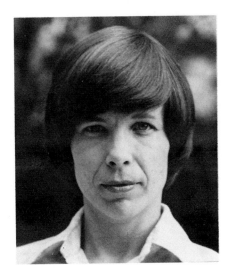

Foreword

The emergence of hand surgery as a specialty and the advances in the science and art of hand surgery since World War II have been truly phenomenal. Societies for surgery of the hand have attracted some of the most skillful and dedicated surgeons and have served as a forum for discussion and criticism, new concepts, and the testing and trial of competing ideas.

At first, this exciting advance in hand surgery was not accompanied by a parallel advance in techniques of conservative and nonoperative management of the hand. Not only has this led to a tendency to operate on patients who might have been better treated conservatively, but many patients who have rightly and properly been operated on have failed to obtain the best results of their surgery because of inadequate or poorly planned preoperative and postoperative management.

It is encouraging to note that just in the last decade interest has surged in what is being called "hand rehabilitation." This term is used to cover the whole range of conservative management of the hand. It represents an area in which the surgeon and therapist work closely together, with each bringing their special experience and expertise to the common problem. Hand rehabilitation centers are multiplying, and a new group, the Society of Hand Therapists, has been formed in association with the American Society for Surgery of the Hand to bring together those physical therapists and occupational therapists who specialize in the hand.

Pioneers in the new movement are Elaine Fess, Karan Gettle, and James Strickland, and their work has concentrated on the neglected field of hand splinting. Little research has been done on the actual effect of externally applied forces on joints and tissues of the hand. Experienced surgeons and therapists have developed an intuitive "feel" for what can be accomplished, but there is little in the literature to assist the young surgeon in what to prescribe or to help a young therapist know the hazards that can turn a good prescription into a harmful application. In this situation, Elaine Fess, Karan Gettle, and James Strickland have put their own experience down on paper and made it available to all of us. It is obvious that they have a great deal of experience. It is also clear that they have gone far beyond the "cookbook" stage of previous splinting manuals. They have researched and studied their subject thoroughly, and we are fortunate indeed to have the result of that study presented so clearly and illustrated so well.

What pleases me most about this book is that it deals first with principles and only then with specific design. It begins with an emphasis on anatomy and topography and then with mechanical principles; after chapters on principles of design and fit and construction, the authors discuss specific splints. In addition, there is a good chapter on specific problems and how to handle them.

It is a measure of how far we still have to go in the science of splinting that the authors do not feel able to recommend actual specific forces by numbers to use in dynamic splints. My own feeling is that the boundary between art and science is numbers. Even in hand surgery we are not yet able to say that a specific tendon should be attached with a tension of 200 grams, so why should we expect a therapist to fix a rubber band at a specific level of tension? One day we will take these extra steps toward precision. When data are available, Elaine Fess, Karan Gettle, and James Strickland will be the first to put it into their next book. They have jumped into a clear position of leadership with this book. I am sure they will stay ahead of each new advance as it comes along.

Paul W. Brand, F.R.C.S.
Clinical Professor of Surgery and Orthopaedics,
Louisiana State University; Chief, Rehabilitation Branch,
United States Public Health Service Hospital,
Carville, Louisiana

Preface

Webster's Unabridged Dictionary describes splints as "rigid or flexible appliances used for the prevention of movement of a joint or for the fixation of displaced or movable parts." However, in current medical practice the boundaries of this definition have been expanded to include a greater variety of devices that not only prevent joint motion but also maintain or enhance it. It is now recognized that such appliances can serve many important roles in the management of disease and injury of the hand. Splints may be employed to prevent deformity of, immobilize, mobilize, position, or protect the wrist and digital joints with the intent of restoring maximum function. Design and construction of splints have ranged from abject simplicity to complex appliances reminiscent of Rube Goldberg contraptions.

Medical science treatises devoted to the management of injuries and disease of the upper extremity have contained illustrations of clever devices designed to prevent or correct deformities. Drawings of some of these devices are shown on pp. x and xi. Interestingly, modern literature has done little more than elaborate on these devices with techniques developed for the simplified preparation of more comfortable splints made possible by the development of new materials. Unfortunately, there has been an appalling lack of a scientific approach to the design and preparation of hand splints. Devices constructed without an adequate understanding of the underlying pathologic conditions of the hand, the realistic goals expected of a given splint, and the mechanics that must be correctly used to achieve these goals will often prove to be failures.

Although many hand splints have been proposed with great concern for individual anatomic and pathologic differences, others are mass produced commercially for application to a wide spectrum of clinical conditions. An appreciation of the enormous variation in hand size and configuration and for the almost endless number of possible conditions that may exist in the upper extremity should lead one to worry about the potential pitfalls of the rote application of such standardized devices.

Although the proper use of hand splints is now considered an essential part of the management of patients with acute or chronic disease or injury of the hand and upper extremity, an approach to the preparation of these splints must be made

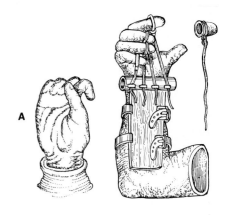

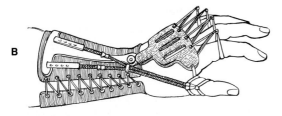

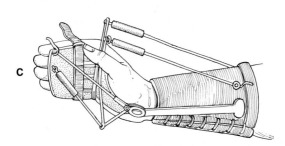

Although these splints initially appear barbaric, close scrutiny reveals that many of the principles employed during the past three centuries for splinting the hand continue to be applicable today.

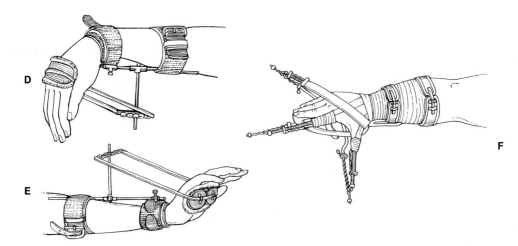

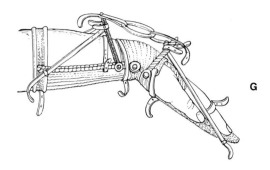

G

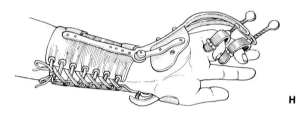

H

A, 1647; B and C, 1869; D and E, 1886; F, 1889; G, 1908; H, 1927; I, 1943; J, 1949. (Modified from Boyes, J. H., editor: Bunnell's surgery of the hand, ed. 5, Philadelphia, 1970, J. B. Lippincott Co.)

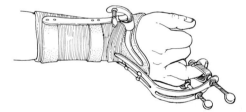

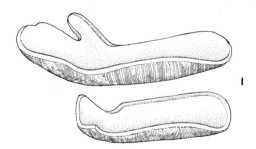

I

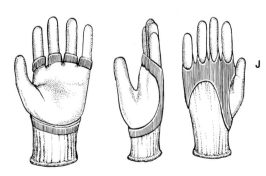

J

with a thorough understanding of the underlying anatomic alterations and the realistic therapeutic considerations – be they medical, surgical, or rehabilitative – that comprise the total treatment program. The patient's management cannot be fragmented into these various components, but requires a close working relationship among patient, surgeon, and therapist to provide an integrated approach that achieves maximum functional benefit. It is not enough for the person engaged in the preparation of a hand splint to create that splint from a prescription supplied at long range by a surgeon who has undertaken the initial management or reconstructive effort of a given hand problem. The insufficient information created by this "communication gap" will almost inevitably lead not only to an incorrectly prepared splint, but also to confusion on the part of the patient and therapist as to the exact goals and realistic expectations of such a device. We cannot overemphasize, therefore, the need for an excellent line of communication between surgeon and therapist, with extensive instruction to the patient not only with regard to splint use, but also to the desired objectives of splinting. Only through this close working relationship can the correct preparation and use of splints be expected.

In *Hand Splinting: Principles and Methods,* we have reviewed the anatomy and kinesiology of the hand to provide a sound, basic understanding of the important underlying structures and their function. We have discussed the mechanical principles that must be employed in the preparation of hand splints. A classification and description of the nomenclature of various splints and splint components is also provided, together with an extensive examination of the principles of splint fit, construction, and design. A breakdown of splint considerations by anatomic area is provided, as well as a review of the use of splints for special problems and the importance of exercise. A survey of the materials and equipment, splint checkout and referral forms, work area examples, and American Society for Surgery of the Hand Clinical Assessment Recommendations are included in the appendices.

Hand Splinting: Principles and Methods is presented in a learning theory hierarchy in which basic principles are discussed and examples given. Once readers progress through the fundamental early chapters, they are provided with the opportunity to use this acquired information by analyzing splints that are incorrectly designed, constructed, or fitted. Immediate feedback is given for each splint so that readers may compare their analysis with ours.

We concede at the onset that a particular splint may not be best for any one clinical situation and that in many cases one may choose from a wide variety of splints to try to accomplish a given therapeutic goal. Nonetheless, it is important for the person preparing the splint to thoroughly understand the exact purpose for the splint being prepared, the necessary mechanics to achieve it, and the available design options. We have attempted to leave these specific splint selection decisions to readers and to simply review the various possibilities, with discussion of the various advantages and disadvantages of each. The philosophy of the book is predicated on the design of individual splints for specific problems from basic splint components. We emphasize that there are no rote splinting solutions to combating pathologic conditions of the hand and that each splint is created on an individual basis using the principles of mechanics, fit, construction, and design. Although we acknowledge a redundancy in the discussion of many of the principles and specific splint considerations, we believe that this approach will provide the best ultimate understanding of the important role of splinting in the management of hand disease and injury.

We gratefully acknowledge the continued help and support our families have given us during the writing of *Hand Splinting: Principles and Methods*. Sherran Schmalfeldt, Geanora Westlake, and Jan Casner deserve recognition for the many hours spent in typing the manuscript. Craig Gosling, Carol Stahl, Joe Demma, and Tom Royhans must be commended for their excellent illustrations and photographs. Special appreciation goes to Richard Dunnipace, Ph.D., for proofreading the mechanics chapter. We also thank Roylan Manufacturing Company, Johnson and Johnson, and Abbey Rents, who generously donated materials for many of the splints illustrated. Finally, we express our admiration and gratitude to the patients of the Hand Rehabilitation Center of Indiana in Indianapolis, without whose assistance this book could not have been written.

Elaine Ewing Fess
Karan S. Gettle
James W. Strickland

Contents

CHAPTER 1

Anatomy and kinesiology of the hand

One cannot expect to adequately participate in the treatment of disorders of the hand and arm without a solid working knowledge of the intricate anatomic and kinesiologic relationships of the upper extremity. The preparation of externally applied splinting devices to the forearm, wrist, and hand necessitates a thorough understanding of and respect for the underlying anatomic structures. Only through comprehension of the normal anatomy of the human hand can one adequately develop an appreciation for the anatomic alterations that accompany injury and disease. It is appropriate, therefore, that the first chapter in a book devoted to hand splinting be concerned with the anatomy and kinesiology of the hand. Since it is impossible in this chapter to review in great detail the enormous amount of literature that has been written about the anatomic, kinesiologic, and biomechanical aspects of the hand, readers are directed to the Bibliography for more extensive reading on these subjects.

The anatomy of the hand must of necessity be approached in a systematic fashion with individual consideration of the osseous structures, joints, musculotendinous units, blood supply, nerve supply, and surface anatomy. However, it is obvious that the systems do not function independently, but that the integrated presence of all these structures is required for normal hand function. In presenting this material, we will stray into the important mechanical and kinesiologic considerations that result from the unique anatomic arrangement of the hand and briefly try to indicate the problems resulting from various forms of pathologic conditions in certain areas. Surface anatomy and a description of the basic patterns of hand function will also be included at the end of this chapter.

OSSEOUS STRUCTURES

The unique arrangement and mobility of the bones of the hand (Fig. 1-1) provide a structural basis for its enormous functional adaptability. The osseous skeleton consists of eight carpal bones divided into two rows: the proximal row articulates with the distal radius and ulna; the distal four carpal bones in turn articulate with the five metacarpals. Two phalanges complete the first metacarpal, or thumb unit, and three phalanges each comprise the index, long, ring, and small fingers. These twenty-seven bones, together with the intricate arrangement of supportive

1

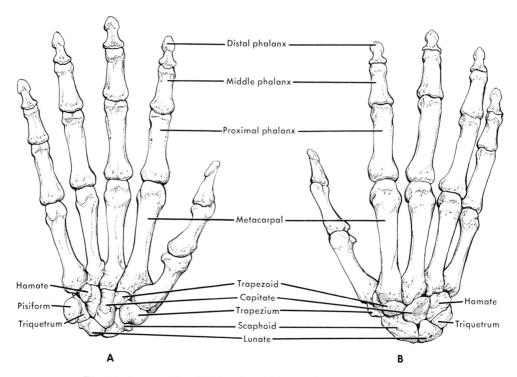

Distal phalanx

Middle phalanx

Proximal phalanx

Metacarpal

Hamate
Pisiform
Triquetrum

Trapezoid
Capitate
Trapezium
Scaphoid
Lunate

Hamate
Triquetrum

A   B

Fig. 1-1. Bones of the right hand. **A,** Volar surface. **B,** Dorsal surface.

ligaments and contractile musculotendinous units, are arranged to provide both mobility and stability to the various joints of the hand. Although the exact anatomic configuration of the bones of the hand need not be memorized in detail, it is important to develop a knowledge of the position and names of the carpal bones, metacarpals, and phalanges and an understanding of their kinesiologic patterns to proceed with the management of many hand problems.

The bones of the hand are arranged in three arches (Fig. 1-2), two of which are transversely oriented and one of which is longitudinal. The proximal transverse arch, the keystone of which is the capitate, lies at the level of the distal part of the carpus and is rigid, whereas the distal transverse arch passing through the metacarpal heads is more mobile. The two transverse arches are connected by the rigid portion of the longitudinal arch consisting of the second and third metacarpals, the index and long fingers distally and the central carpus proximally. The longitudinal arch is completed by the individual digital rays, and the mobility of the first, fourth, and fifth rays around the second and third allows the palm to flatten or cup itself in response to objects of various sizes and shapes.

To a large extent the intrinsic muscles of the hand are responsible for changes in the configuration of the osseous arches, and collapse in the arch system resulting from injury to the osseous skeleton or paralysis of these intrinsic muscles can contribute to severe disability and deformity. Flatt (1972) has pointed out that grasp

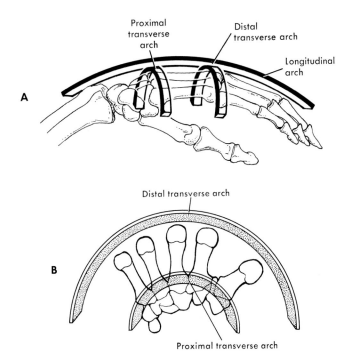

Fig. 1-2. A, Skeletal arches of the hand. The proximal transverse arch passes through the distal carpus; the distal transverse arch, through the metacarpal heads. The longitudinal arch is made up of the four digital rays and the carpus proximally. **B,** Proximal and distal transverse arches.

is dependent on the integrity of the mobile longitudinal arches and that, when destruction at the carpometacarpal joint, metacarpophalangeal joint, or proximal interphalangeal joint interrupts the integrity of these arches, crippling deformity may result.

JOINTS

The multiple complex articulations between the distal radius and ulna, the eight carpal bones, and the metacarpal bases comprise the wrist joint, whose proximal position makes it the functional key to the motion at the more distal digital joints of the hand. The proximal carpal row, consisting of the scaphoid (navicular), lunate, triquetrum, and pisiform, articulates distally with the trapezium, trapezoid, capitate, and hamate, and a definite complex pattern of motion among these small bones and their proximal and distal articulations is present. The stability as well as the range of motion of the wrist is governed by the strong ligamentous support system that exists on both the volar and dorsal surfaces. Radial and ulnar collateral ligaments connecting the radial styloid to the radial side of the scaphoid and trapezium and the ulnar styloid to the triquetrum, pisiform, and triangular fibrocartilage provides strong lateral support and restraint. In addition, radio-

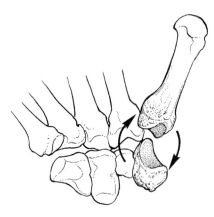

Fig. 1-3. Saddle-shaped carpometacarpal joint of the thumb. A wide range of motion *(arrows)* is permitted by the configuration of this joint.

carpal and intracarpal ligaments exercise control over dorsal and volar flexion motions.

Volar flexion takes place to a greater extent in the radiocarpal joint and secondarily in the midcarpal joint, whereas dorsiflexion occurs primarily at the midcarpal joint and only secondarily in the radiocarpal articulation. It is believed that radial deviation is produced in the midcarpal joint and ulnar deviation at the radiocarpal joint.

The articulation between the base of the first metacarpal and the trapezium (Fig. 1-3) is a highly mobile joint with a configuration thought to be similar to that of a saddle. The base of the first metacarpal is concave in the anteroposterior plane and convex in the lateral plane, with a reciprocal concavity in the lateral plane and an anteroposterior convexity on the opposing surface of the trapezium. This arrangement allows for the positioning of the thumb in a wide arc of motion (Fig. 1-4), including flexion, extension, abduction, adduction, and opposition. The ligamentous arrangement about this joint, while permitting the wide circumduction, continues to provide stability at the extremes of motion, allowing the thumb to be brought into a variety of positions for pinch and grasp, but maintaining its stability during these functions. A similar articulation is formed by the ulnar half of the hamate and the fifth metacarpal base, allowing for more motion at this joint than is permitted at the bases of the index, long, and ring fingers.

The metacarpophalangeal joints of the fingers are diarthrodial joints with motion permitted in three planes and combinations thereof (Fig. 1-5). The cartilaginous surfaces of the metacarpal head and the bases of the proximal phalanges are enclosed in a complex apparatus consisting of the joint capsule, collateral ligaments, and the anterior fibrocartilage or volar plate (Fig. 1-6). The capsule extends from the borders of the base of the proximal phalanx proximally to the head of the metacarpals beyond the cartilaginous joint surface. The collateral ligaments, which reinforce the capsule on each side of the metacarpophalangeal joints, run from the dorsolateral side of the metacarpal head to the volar lateral side of the proximal phalanges. These ligaments form two bundles, the more central of which is referred to as the *cord portion of the collateral ligament* and inserts into the

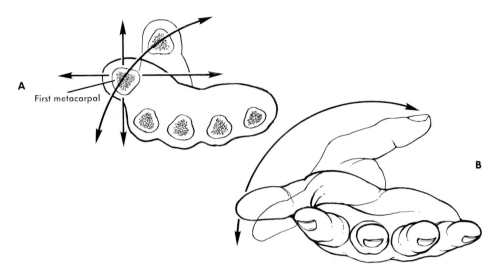

Fig. 1-4. A, Multiple planes of motion *(arrows)* that occur at the carpometacarpal joint of the thumb. **B,** The thumb moves *(arrow)* from a position of adduction against the second metacarpal to a position of extension abduction away from the hand and fingers and can then be rotated into positions of opposition and flexion.

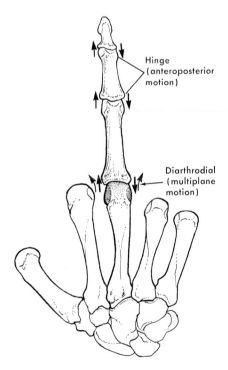

Fig. 1-5. Joints of the phalanges. The diarthrodial configuration of the metacarpophalangeal joint permits motion in multiple planes, whereas the biconcave-convex hinge configuration of the interphalangeal joints restricts motion to the anteroposterior plane.

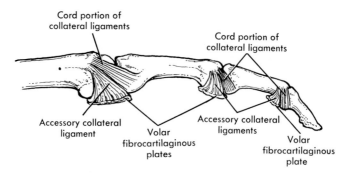

Fig. 1-6. Ligamentous structures of the digital joints. The collateral ligaments of the meta-carpophalangeal and interdigital joints are composed of a strong cord portion with bony origin and insertion. The more volarly placed accessory collateral ligaments originate from the proximal bone and insert into the volar fibrocartilaginous plate. The volar plates have strong distal attachments to resist extension forces.

side of the proximal phalanx; the more volar portion joins the palmar plate and is termed the *accessory collateral ligament.* These collateral ligaments are some-what loose with the metacarpophalangeal joint in extension, allowing for con-siderable "play" in the side-to-side motion of the digits (Fig. 1-7). With the metacarpophalangeal joints in full flexion, however, the cam configuration of the metacarpal head tightens the collateral ligaments and limits lateral mobility of the digits. This alteration in tension becomes an important factor in immobiliza-tion of the metacarpophalangeal joints for any length of time, since the secondary shortening of the laxed collateral ligaments that may occur when these joints are immobilized in extension will result in severe limitation of metacarpophalan-geal joint flexion by these structures.

The volar fibrocartilaginous plate on the palmar side of the metacarpophalan-geal joint is firmly attached to the base of the proximal phalanx and loosely at-tached to the anterior surface of the neck of the metacarpal by means of the joint capsule at the neck of the metacarpal. This arrangement allows the volar plate to slide proximally during metacarpophalangeal joint flexion. The flexor ten-dons pass along a groove on the front of the plate, and the volar plates are con-nected by the transverse intermetacarpal ligament, which extends from the index to the fifth finger.

The metacarpophalangeal joint of the thumb differs from the others in that the head of the first metacarpal is flatter, and its cartilaginous surface does not extend as far laterally or posteriorly. Two small sesamoid bones are also adjacent to this joint, and the ligamentous structure differs somewhat. A few degrees of abduction and rotation are permitted by the ligament arrangement of the metacarpopha-langeal joint at the thumb, which is of considerable functional importance in delicate precision functions.

The digital interphalangeal joints are hinge joints (Fig. 1-5) and, like the meta-carpophalangeal joints, have capsular and ligamentous enclosure. The articular surface of the proximal phalangeal head is convex in the anteroposterior plane

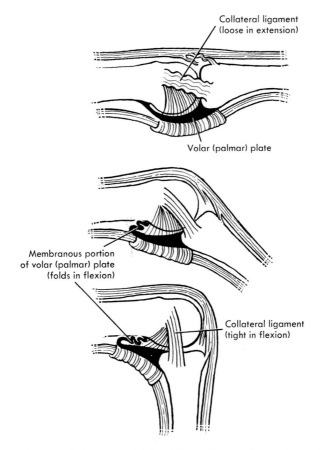

Collateral ligament
(loose in extension)

Volar (palmar) plate

Membranous portion
of volar (palmar) plate
(folds in flexion)

Collateral ligament
(tight in flexion)

Fig. 1-7. At the metacarpophalangeal joint level the collateral ligaments are loose in extension but become tightened in flexion. The proximal membranous portion of the palmar plate moves proximally to accommodate for flexion. (Modified from Wynn Parry, C. B., et al.: Rehabilitation of the hand, ed. 3, London, 1973, Butterworth & Co. [Publishers], Ltd.)

with a depression in the middle between the two condyles, which articulates with the phalanx distal to it. The bases of the middle and distal phalanges appear as a concave surface with an elevated ridge dividing two concave depressions. A cord portion of the collateral ligament and an accessory collateral ligament are present, and the collateral ligaments run on each side of the joint from the posterolateral aspect of the proximal phalanx in a volar and lateral direction to insert into the distally placed phalanx and its fibrocartilage plate (Fig. 1-8). A strong fibrocartilaginous (volar) plate is also present, and the collateral ligaments of the proximal and distal interphalangeal joints are tightest with the joints in near full extension.

The stability of the proximal interphalangeal joint is assured by a three-sided supporting cradle produced by the junction of the volar plate with the base of the middle phalanx and the accessory collateral ligament structures (Fig. 1-8). The confluence of ligaments is strongly anchored by proximal and lateral extensions

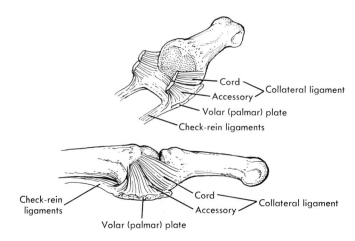

Fig. 1-8. Strong, three-sided ligamentous support system of the proximal interphalangeal joint with cord and accessory collateral ligaments and the fibrocartilaginous plate, which is anchored proximally by the check-rein ligamentous attachment. (Modified from Eaton, R. G.: Joint injuries of the hand, Springfield, Ill., 1971, Charles C Thomas, Publisher.)

referred to as the *check-rein ligaments*. This system has been described as a three-dimensional hinge that results in remarkable volar and lateral restraint.

A wide range of pathologic conditions may result from the interruption of the supportive ligament systems of the intercarpal or digital joints. At the wrist level, interruption of key radiocarpal or intercarpal ligaments may result in occult patterns of wrist instability that are often difficult to diagnose and treat. In the digits, disruption of the collateral ligaments or the fibrocartilaginous volar plates will produce joint laxity or deformity, which is more obvious. Rupture or attenuation of these supporting structures may result not only from trauma, but may also occur more insidiously with chronic disease processes such as arthritis.

MUSCLES AND TENDONS

The muscles acting on the hand can be grouped as extrinsic, when their muscle bellies are in the forearm, or intrinsic, when the muscles originate distal to the wrist joint. It is important to thoroughly understand both systems. Although their contribution to hand function is distinctly different, the integrated function of both systems is important to the satisfactory performance of the hand in a wide variety of tasks. A schematic representation of the origin and insertion of the extrinsic flexor and extensor muscle tendon units of the hand is provided in Figs. 1-9 to 1-13. The important nerve supply to each muscle group will be reviewed in these figures and again when discussing the nerve supply to the upper extremity.

Extrinsic muscles

The extrinsic flexor muscles (Fig. 1-9) of the forearm form a prominent mass on the medial side of the upper part of the forearm: the most superficial group is

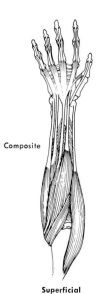

Composite

Superficial

Fig. 1-9. Extrinsic flexor muscles of the arm and hand. (Dark areas represent origins and insertions of muscles.) (Modified from Marble, H. C.: The hand, a manual and atlas for the general surgeon, Philadelphia, 1960, W. B. Saunders Co.)

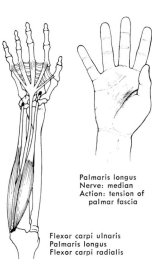

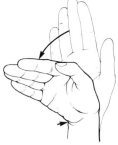

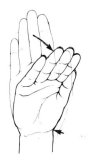

Palmaris longus
Nerve: median
Action: tension of
   palmar fascia

Flexor carpi ulnaris
Nerve: ulnar
Action: flexion of wrist;
   ulnar deviation of
   hand

Flexor carpi radialis
Nerve: median
Action: flexion of wrist;
   radial deviation
   of hand

Flexor carpi ulnaris
Palmaris longus
Flexor carpi radialis

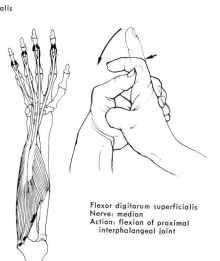

Flexor digitorum superficialis
Nerve: median
Action: flexion of proximal
   interphalangeal joint

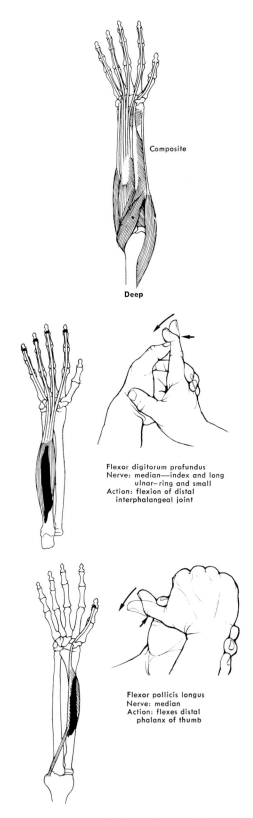

Composite

Deep

Flexor digitorum profundus
Nerve: median—index and long
            ulnar–ring and small
Action: flexion of distal
       interphalangeal joint

Flexor pollicis longus
Nerve: median
Action: flexes distal
      phalanx of thumb

Fig. 1-9. For legend see p. 9.

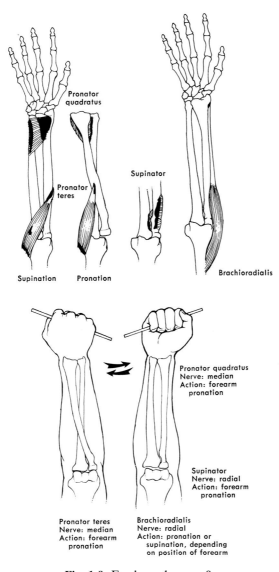

Fig. 1-9. For legend see p. 9.

comprised by the pronator teres, the flexor carpi radialis, the flexor carpi ulnaris, and the palmaris longus; the intermediate group, by the flexor digitorum superficialis; and the deep extrinsics, by the flexor digitorum profundus and the flexor pollicis longus. The pronator, palmaris, wrist flexors, and superficialis tendons arise from the area about the medial epicondyle, the ulnar collateral ligament of the elbow, and the medial aspect of the coronoid process. The flexor pollicis longus originates from the entire middle third of the volar surface of the radius and the adjacent interosseous membrane, and the flexor digitorum profundus originates deep to the other muscles of the forearm from the proximal two thirds of the ulna on the volar and medial side. The deepest layer of the volar forearm is completed distally by the pronator quadratus muscle.

The flexor carpi radialis tendon inserts on the base of the second metacarpal, whereas the flexor carpi ulnaris shares its insertion over the pisiform and fifth metacarpal base. The superficialis tendons lie on the volar side of the profundus tendons as far as the digital bases, where they bifurcate and wrap around the profundi to insert on the proximal aspect of the middle phalanges. The profundi continue through the superficialis decussation to insert on the base of the distal phalanges, whereas the flexor pollicis longus inserts on the base of the distal phalanx of the thumb.

At the wrist the nine long flexor tendons enter the carpal tunnel beneath the protective roof of the deep transverse carpal ligament in company with the median nerve. In this canal the common profundus tendon to the long, ring, and small fingers divides into the individual tendons that fan out distally and proceed toward the distal phalanges of these digits (Fig. 1-10). At approximately the level of the distal palmar crease the paired profundus and superficialis tendons to the index, long, ring, and small fingers and the flexor pollicis longus to the thumb enter the individual flexor sheaths that house them throughout the remainder of their digital course. These sheaths with their predictable annular pulley arrangement (Fig. 1-11) serve not only as a protective housing for the flexor tendons, but also provide a smooth gliding surface by virtue of their synovial lining and an efficient mechanism to hold the tendons close to the digital bone and joints. There is an increasing recognition that disruption of this valuable pulley system can produce substantial mechanical alterations in digital function, resulting in imbalance and deformity.

Extension of the wrist and fingers is produced by the extrinsic extensor muscle tendon system, which consists of the two radial wrist extensors, the extensor carpi ulnaris, the extensor digitorum communis, and the extensor digiti quinti proprius (extensor digiti minimi) (Fig. 1-12). These muscles originate in common from the lateral epicondyle and the lateral epicondylar ridge and from a small area posterior to the radial notch of the ulna. The brachioradialis originates from the epicondylar line proximal to the lateral epicondyle, and, because it inserts on the distal radius, it does not truly contribute to wrist or digit motion. The extensor carpi radialis longus and brevis insert proximally on the bases of the second and

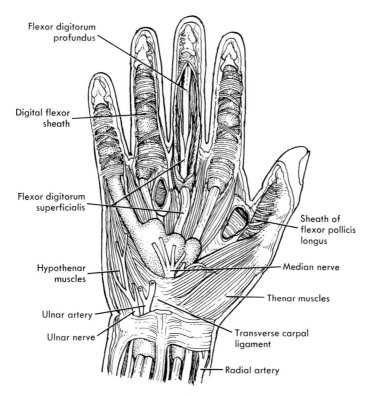

Flexor digitorum profundus

Digital flexor sheath

Flexor digitorum superficialis

Hypothenar muscles

Ulnar artery

Ulnar nerve

Sheath of flexor pollicis longus

Median nerve

Thenar muscles

Transverse carpal ligament

Radial artery

Fig. 1-10. Flexor tendons in the palm and digits. Fibro-osseous digital sheaths with their pulley arrangement are shown, as is a division of the superficialis tendon about the profundus in the proximal portion of the sheath.

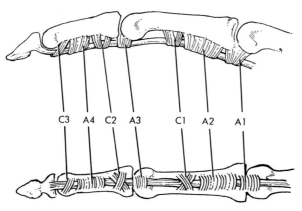

C3   A4   C2   A3   C1   A2   A1

Fig. 1-11. Pulley system of the digits. (Modified from Doyle, J. R., and Blythe, W.: The finger flexor tendon sheath and pulleys: anatomy and reconstruction. In American Academy of Orthopaedic Surgeons: Symposium on Tendon Surgery in the Hand, St. Louis, 1975, The C. V. Mosby Co.)

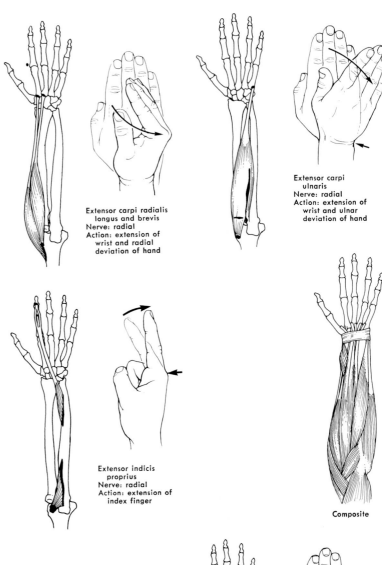

Extensor carpi radialis
longus and brevis
Nerve: radial
Action: extension of
wrist and radial
deviation of hand

Extensor carpi
ulnaris
Nerve: radial
Action: extension of
wrist and ulnar
deviation of hand

Extensor indicis
proprius
Nerve: radial
Action: extension of
index finger

Composite

Fig. 1-12. Extensor muscles of the forearm and hand. (Modified from Marble, H. C.: The hand, a manual and atlas for the general surgeon, Philadelphia, 1960, W. B. Saunders Co.)

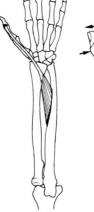
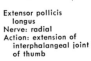

Extensor pollicis
longus
Nerve: radial
Action: extension of
interphalangeal joint
of thumb

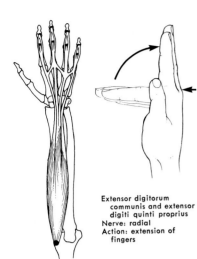

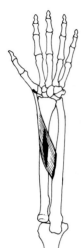

Extensor digitorum
  communis and extensor
  digiti quinti proprius
Nerve: radial
Action: extension of
  fingers

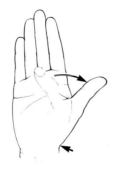

Abductor pollicis
  longus
Nerve: radial
Action: abduction of thumb

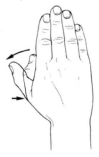

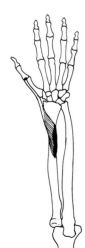

Extensor pollicis brevis
Nerve: radial
Action: extension of
  metacarpophalangeal
  joint of thumb

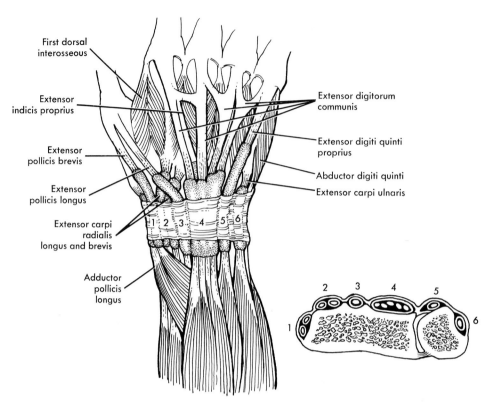

Fig. 1-13. Arrangement of the extensor tendons in the compartments of the wrist. (Modified from Lampe, E. W.: Surgical anatomy of the hand. In Clinical symposia, New York, 1969, CIBA Pharmaceutical Co., Division of CIBA-GEIGY Corp.; illustrated by F. H. Netter.)

third metacarpals, respectively, and the extensor carpi ulnaris inserts on the base of the fifth metacarpal. The long digital extensors terminate by insertions on the base of the middle phalanges after receiving and giving fibers to the intrinsic tendons to form the lateral bands that are destined to insert on the bases of the distal phalanx. Digital extension, therefore, results from a combination of the contribution of both the extrinsic and intrinsic extensor systems. The extensor pollicis longus and brevis tendons, together with the abductor pollicis longus, originate from the dorsal forearm and, by virtue of their respective insertions into the distal phalanx, proximal phalanx, and first metacarpal of the thumb, provide extension at all three levels. The extensor pollicis longus approaches the thumb obliquely around a small bony tubercle on the dorsal radius (Lister's tubercle) and therefore functions not only as an extensor but as a strong secondary adductor of the thumb. The extensor indicis proprius also originates more distally from an area near the origin of the thumb extensor and long abductor. The extensor digiti quinti proprius arises near the lateral epicondyle to occupy a superficial position on the dorsum of the forearm with its tendon inserting into the middle phalanx of the small finger.

At the wrist, the extensor tendons are divided into six dorsal compartments (Fig. 1-13). The first compartment consists of the tendons of the abductor pollicis longus and extensor pollicis brevis, and the second compartment houses the two radial wrist extensors, the extensor carpi radialis longus and brevis. The third compartment is composed of the tendon of the extensor pollicis longus, and the fourth compartment allows passage of the four communis extensor tendons and the extensor indicis proprius tendon. The extensor digiti quinti proprius travels through the fifth dorsal compartment, and the sixth houses the extensor carpi ulnaris.

Intrinsic muscles

The important intrinsic musculature of the hand can be divided into muscles comprising the thenar eminence, those comprising the hypothenar eminence, and the remaining muscles between the two groups (Fig. 1-14). The muscles of the thenar eminence consist of the abductor pollicis brevis, the flexor pollicis brevis, and the opponens pollicis, which originate in common from the transverse carpal ligament and the scaphoid and trapezium bones. The abductor brevis inserts into the radial side of the proximal phalanx and the radial wing tendon of the thumb, as does the flexor pollicis brevis, whereas the opponens inserts into the whole radial side of the first metacarpal.

The flexor pollicis brevis has a superficial portion that is innervated by the median nerve and a deep portion that arises from the ulnar side of the first meta-carpal and is often innervated by the ulnar nerve. The hypothenar eminence in a similar manner is made up of the abductor digiti quinti, the flexor digiti quinti brevis, and the opponens digiti quinti, which originate primarily from the pisiform bone and the pisohamate ligament and insert into the joint capsule of the fifth metacarpophalangeal joint, the ulnar side of the base of the proximal phalanx of the fifth finger, and the ulnar border of the aponeurosis of this digit. The strong thenar musculature is responsible for the ability to position the thumb to meet the adjacent digits for pinch and grasp functions, whereas the hypothenar group allows a similar but less pronounced rotation of the fifth metacarpal.

Of the seven interosseous muscles (Fig. 1-15, *A*), four are considered in the dorsal group (Fig. 1-15, *B*), and three as volar interossei (Fig. 1-15, *C*). The dorsal interossei originate from the adjacent sides of the metacarpal bones, and, because of their bipinnate nature with multiple individual muscle bellies, separate insertions into the tubercle and the lateral aspect of the proximal phalanges and into the extensor expansion are provided. The more volarly placed palmar interossei (Fig. 1-15, *C*) have similar insertions and origins and are responsible for adducting the digits together, as opposed to the spreading or abducting function of the dorsal interossei. In addition, four lumbrical tendons (Fig. 1-16, *A*) arising from the radial side of the palmar portion of the flexor digitorum profundus tendons pass

Text continued on p. 22.

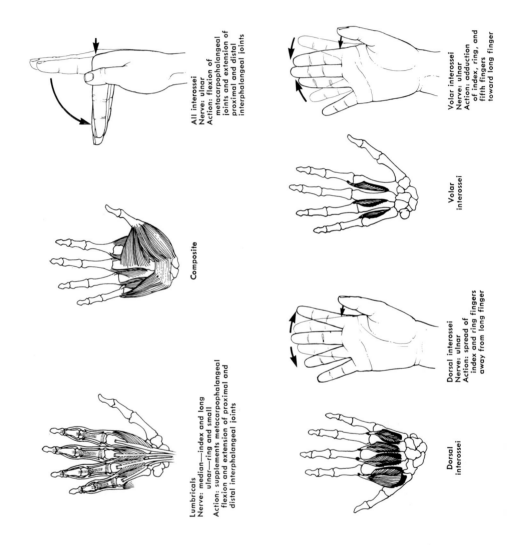

All interossei
Nerve: ulnar
Action: flexion of metacarpophalangeal joints and extension of proximal and distal interphalangeal joints

Composite

Lumbricals
Nerve: median—index and long ulnar—ring and small
Action: supplements metacarpophalangeal flexion and extension of proximal and distal interphalangeal joints

Volar interossei
Nerve: ulnar
Action: adduction of index, ring, and fifth fingers toward long finger

Volar interossei

Dorsal interossei
Nerve: ulnar
Action: spread of index and ring fingers away from long finger

Dorsal interossei

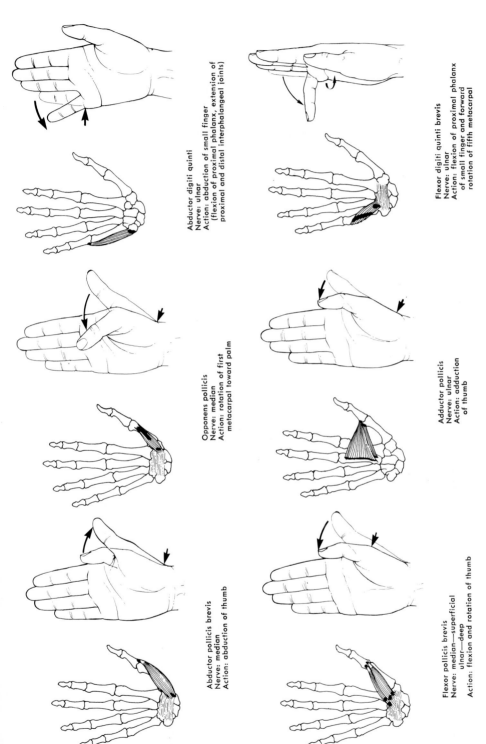

Abductor digiti quinti
Nerve: ulnar
Action: abduction of small finger
  (flexion of proximal phalanx, extension of
  proximal and distal interphalangeal joints)

Flexor digiti quinti brevis
Nerve: ulnar
Action: flexion of proximal phalanx
  of small finger and forward
  rotation of fifth metacarpal

Opponens pollicis
Nerve: median
Action: rotation of first
  metacarpal toward palm

Adductor pollicis
Nerve: ulnar
Action: adduction
  of thumb

Abductor pollicis brevis
Nerve: median
Action: abduction of thumb

Flexor pollicis brevis
Nerve: median—superficial
  ulnar—deep
Action: flexion and rotation of thumb

Fig. 1-14. Intrinsic muscles of the hand. (Modified from Marble, H. C.: The hand, a manual and atlas for the general surgeon, Philadelphia, 1960, W. B. Saunders Co.)

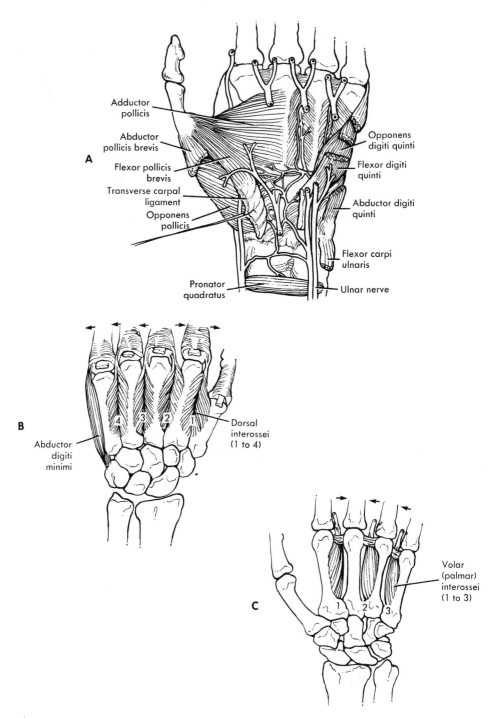

Fig. 1-15. Position and function of the intrinsic muscles of the hand. (Modified from Lampe, E. W.: Surgical anatomy of the hand. In Clinical symposia, New York, 1969, CIBA Pharmaceutical Co., Division of CIBA-GEIGY Corp.; illustrated by F. H. Netter.)

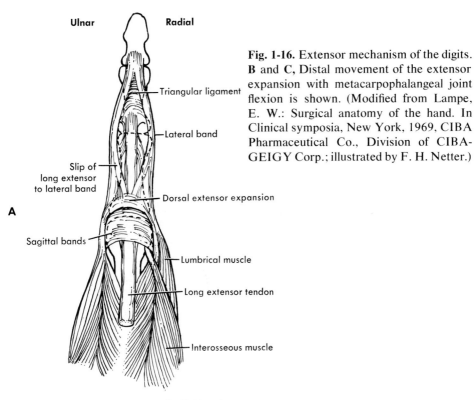

Ulnar   Radial

Triangular ligament

Lateral band

Slip of
long extensor
to lateral band

A

Dorsal extensor expansion

Sagittal bands

Lumbrical muscle

Long extensor tendon

Interosseous muscle

Fig. 1-16. Extensor mechanism of the digits. B and C, Distal movement of the extensor expansion with metacarpophalangeal joint flexion is shown. (Modified from Lampe, E. W.: Surgical anatomy of the hand. In Clinical symposia, New York, 1969, CIBA Pharmaceutical Co., Division of CIBA-GEIGY Corp.; illustrated by F. H. Netter.)

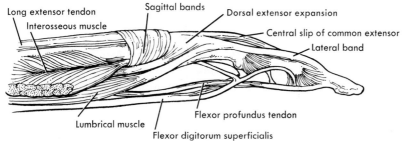

Long extensor tendon   Sagittal bands   Dorsal extensor expansion

Interosseous muscle   Central slip of common extensor

Lateral band

B

Lumbrical muscle

Flexor profundus tendon

Flexor digitorum superficialis

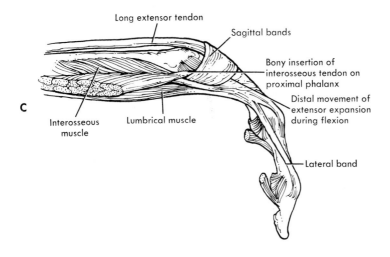

Long extensor tendon   Sagittal bands

Bony insertion of
interosseous tendon on
proximal phalanx

Distal movement of
extensor expansion
during flexion

C

Interosseous
muscle   Lumbrical muscle

Lateral band

through their individual canals on the radial side of the digits to provide an additional contribution to the complex extensor assemblage of the digits. The arrangement of the extensor mechanism, including the transverse sagittal band fibers at the metacarpophalangeal joint and the components of the extensor hood mechanism that gain fibers from both the extrinsic and intrinsic tendons, can be seen in Fig. 1-16, *B* and *C*.

An oversimplification of the function of the intrinsic musculature in the digits would be that they provide strong flexion at the metacarpophalangeal joints and extension at the proximal and distal interphalangeal joints. The lumbrical tendons, by virtue of their origin from the flexor profundi and insertion into the digital extensor mechanism, function as a governor between the two systems, resulting in a loosening of the antagonistic profundus tendon during interphalangeal joint extension. The interossei are further responsible for spreading and closing of the fingers and, together with the extrinsic flexor and extensor tendons, are invaluable to digital balance. A composite, well-integrated pattern of digital flexion and extension is reliant on the smooth performance of both systems, and a loss of intrinsic function will result in severe deformity.

Perhaps the most important intrinsic muscle, the adductor pollicis (Fig. 1-15, *A*), originates from the third metacarpal and inserts on the ulnar side of the base of the proximal phalanx of the thumb and into the ulnar wing expansion of the extensor mechanism. This muscle, by virtue of its strong adducting influence on the thumb and its stabilizing effect on the first metacarpophalangeal joint, functions together with the first dorsal interosseous to provide strong pinch. The adductor pollicis, deep head of the flexor pollicis brevis, ulnar two lumbricals, and all interossei, as well as the hypothenar muscle group, are innervated by the ulnar nerve. Loss of ulnar nerve function has a profound influence on hand function.

Muscle balance

When there is normal resting tone in the extrinsic and intrinsic muscle groups of the forearm and hand, the wrist and digital joints will be maintained in a balanced position. With the forearm midway between pronation and supination, the wrist dorsiflexed, and the digits in moderate flexion, the hand is in the optimum position from which to function.

It may be seen that muscles are usually arranged about joints in pairs so that each musculotendinous unit has at least one antagonistic muscle to balance the involved joint. To a large extent the wrist is the key joint and has a strong influence on the long extrinsic muscle performance at the digital level. Maximal digital flexion strength is facilitated by dorsiflexion of the wrist, which lessens the effective amplitude of the antagonistic extensor tendons while maximizing the contractural force of the digital flexors. Conversely, a posture of wrist flexion will markedly weaken grasping power.

At the digital level, metacarpophalangeal joint flexion is a combination of extrinsic flexor power supplemented by the contribution of the intrinsic muscles, whereas proximal interphalangeal joint extension results from a combination of extrinsic extensor and intrinsic muscle power. At the distal interphalangeal joint the intrinsic muscles provide a majority of the extensor power necessary to balance the antagonistic flexor digitorum profundus tendon.

The distance that a tendon moves when its muscle contracts is defined as the amplitude of the tendon and has been measured in numerous studies. In actuality the effective amplitude of any muscle will be limited by the motion permitted by the joint or joints on which its tendon acts. It has been suggested that the amplitude of wrist movers (flexor carpi ulnaris, flexor carpi radialis, extensor carpus radialis longus, extensor carpi radialis brevis, and extensor carpi ulnaris), is approximately 30 mm with the amplitude of finger extensors averaging 50 mm: the thumb flexor, 50 mm; and the finger flexors 70 mm. Although these amplitudes have been thought to be important considerations when deciding on appropriate tendon transfers, Brand (1974) has shown that the potential excursion of a given tendon such as the extensor carpi radialis longus may be considerably greater than the excursion which was required to produce full motion of the joints on which it acted in its original position.

Efforts have been made to determine the power of individual forearm and hand muscles, and a formula based on the physiologic cross section is generally accepted as the best method for determining this value. The number of fibers in cross section determines the absolute muscle power of a given muscle, whereas the force of muscle action times the distance or amplitude of a given muscle determines the work capacity of the muscle. Therefore, a large extrinsic muscle with relatively long fibers such as the flexor digitorum profundus is found to be capable of much more work than is a muscle with shorter fibers such as a wrist extensor. Table 1 is an indicator of the work capacities of the various forearm muscles. It can be seen that the flexor digitorum profundus and superficialis have a significantly greater

Table 1. Work capacity of muscles*

Muscle	mkg
Flexor carpi radialis	0.8
Extensor carpi radialis longus	1.1
Extensor carpi radialis brevis	0.9
Extensor carpi ulnaris	1.1
Abductor pollicis longus	0.1
Flexor pollicis longus	1.2
Flexor digitorum profundus	4.5
Flexor digitorum sublimis (superficialis)	4.8
Brachioradialis	1.9
Flexor carpi ulnaris	2.0
Pronator teres	1.2
Palmaris longus	0.1
Extensor pollicis longus	0.1
Extensor digitorum communis	1.7

*From Von Lanz, T., and Wachsmuth, W.: Praktische anatomie. In Boyes, J. H., editor: Bunnell's surgery of the hand, ed. 5, Philadelphia, 1970, J. B. Lippincott Co.

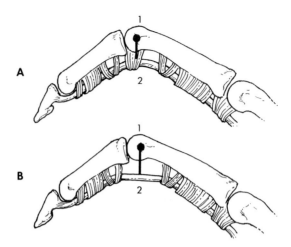

Fig. 1-17. A, The moment arm (*1* and *2*) of a musculotendinous unit is the perpendicular distance between the tendon and the axis of the joint. **B,** A lengthening of the moment arm occurs when the restraining effect of the digital pulley is removed and the tendon is allowed to "bowstring" away from the joint, substantially increasing its angulatory effect at that joint.

work capacity than do the remaining extrinsic muscles. The abductor pollicis longus, palmaris longus, extensor pollicis longus, extensor carpi radialis brevis, and flexor carpi radialis have less than one fourth the capacity of these muscles.

Several mechanical considerations are important in understanding the effect of a muscle on a given joint. The moment arm of a particular muscle is the perpendicular distance between the muscle or its tendon and the axis of the joint. The greater the displacement of an unrestrained tendon from the joint on which it acts, the greater will be the angulatory effect created by the increased length of the moment arm. Therefore, a tendon positioned close to a given joint either by position of the joint or by a restraining pulley will have a much shorter moment arm than will a tendon that is allowed to displace away from the joint (Fig. 1-17).

In simplifying the biomechanics of musculotendinous function, Brand (1974) has emphasized that the "moment" of a given muscle is the power of the muscle to turn a joint on its axis and is determined by multiplying the strength (tension) of the muscle by the length of the moment arm. Again, it can be seen that the distance of tendon displacement away from the joint is the critical factor and that it does not matter where the tendon insertion lies. The importance of the various anatomic restraints on the extrinsic musculotendinous units at the wrist and in the digits is magnified by these mechanical factors.

NERVE SUPPLY

In considering the nerve supply to the forearm, hand, and wrist, it is important to realize that these nerves are a direct continuation of the brachial plexus and that at least a working knowledge of the multiple ramifications of the plexus is

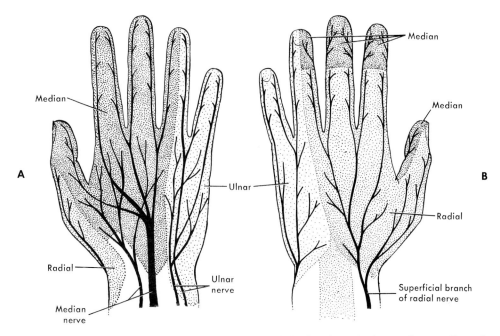

Fig. 1-18. Cutaneous distribution of the nerves of the hand. **A,** Volar surface. **B,** Dorsal surface.

necessary if one is to fully appreciate the more distal motor and sensory contributions of the nerves of the upper extremity. Injuries at either the spinal cord or plexus level or to the major peripheral nerves in the upper extremity result in a substantial functional impairment for which splinting may be necessary.

The median, ulnar, and radial nerves, as well as the terminal course of the musculocutaneous, are responsible for the sensory and motor transmission to the forearm, wrist, and hand. The superficial sensory distribution is shared by the median, radial, and ulnar nerves in a fairly constant pattern (Fig. 1-18). This chapter will be concerned with the most frequent distribution of these nerves, although it is acknowledged that variations are common.

The palmar side of the hand from the thumb to a line passed longitudinally from the tip of the ring finger to the wrist receives sensory innervation from the median nerve. The remainder of the palm as well as the ulnar half of the ring finger and the entire small finger receives sensory innervation from the ulnar nerve. On the dorsal side the ulnar nerve, distribution again includes the ulnar half of the dorsal hand and the ring and small fingers, whereas the radial side is supplied by the superficial branch of the radial nerve. Some innervation to an area distal to the proximal interphalangeal joints is supplied by the volar digital nerves originating from the median nerve. The area around the dorsum of the thumb over the metacarpophalangeal joint is frequently supplied by the end branches of the lateral antebrachial cutaneous nerve.

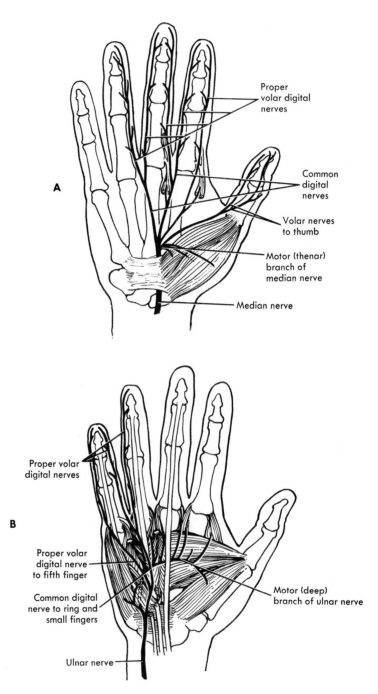

Proper
volar digital
nerves

Common
digital
nerves

Volar nerves
to thumb

Motor (thenar)
branch of
median nerve

Median nerve

A

Proper volar
digital nerves

B

Proper volar
digital nerve
to fifth finger

Common digital
nerve to ring and
small fingers

Motor (deep)
branch of ulnar nerve

Ulnar nerve

Fig. 1-19. Distribution of the median (**A**) and ulnar (**B**) nerves in the palm.

The extrinsic and intrinsic musculature of the forearm and hand is supplied by the median, ulnar, and radial nerves (Fig. 1-19). The long wrist and digital flexors, with the exception of the flexor carpi ulnaris and the profundi to the ring and small fingers, are all supplied by the median nerve. The pronators of the forearm and the muscles of the thenar eminence, with the exception of the deep head of the flexor pollicis brevis and the adductor pollicis, which are innervated by the ulnar nerve, are also supplied by the median nerve. All muscles of the hypothenar eminence, all interossei, the third and fourth lumbrical muscles, the deep head of the flexor pollicis brevis, the adductor pollicis brevis, as well as the flexor carpi ulnaris and ulnar profundi, are supplied by the ulnar nerve. The radial nerve supplies all long extensors of the hand and wrist as well as the long abductor and short extensor of the thumb and the brachioradialis.

When considering sensibility, one should remember that the hand is an extremely important organ for the detection and transmission to the brain of information relating to the size, weight, texture, and temperature of objects with which it comes in contact. The types of cutaneous sensation have been defined as touch, pain, hot, and cold. Although most of the nervous tissue in the skin is found in the dermal network, smaller branches course through the subcutaneous tissue following blood vessels. Several types of sensory receptors have been described, and in most areas of the hand there is an interweaving of nerve fibers that allows each area to receive nerve input from several sources. In addition, deep sensibility from nerve endings in muscles and tendons is important in the recognition of joint position.

The high interruption of the median nerve above the elbow will result in a paralysis of the flexor carpi radialis, the flexor digitorum superficialis, the flexor pollicis longus, the profundi to the index and long fingers, and the lumbricals to the index and long fingers. In addition, pronation will be weakened as a result of the loss of innervation of both the pronator teres and quadratus muscles, and most importantly, the patient will lose the ability to oppose the thumb because of paralysis of the median nerve–innervated thenar muscle group. A more distal interruption of the median nerve at the wrist level will produce loss of opposition, and both lesions will result in a critical impairment of sensation in the important distribution of that nerve to the volar aspect of the thumb, index, long, and radial half of the ring finger.

High ulnar nerve interruption will produce paralysis of the flexor carpi ulnaris, the flexor profundi and lumbricals to the ring and small fingers, and, most importantly, the interossei, adductor pollicis brevis, and deep head of the flexor pollicis brevis. The resulting loss of the antagonistic flexion at the metacarpophalangeal joints of the ring and small fingers will permit hyperextension at this level by the unopposed long extensor tendons, often resulting in a claw deformity. The loss of the strong adducting and stabilizing influence of the adductor pollicis combined with the paralysis of the first dorsal interosseous muscle will result in profound weakness of pinch and produce a collapse deformity of the thumb, necessitating interphalangeal joint hyperflexion for pinch (Froment's sign). More distal lesions of the ulnar nerve will also result in claw deformity, with the profundi function of the ring and small fingers being spared. Sensory loss following ulnar nerve interruption involves the volar ring (ulnar half) and small fingers.

Radial nerve lesions at or proximal to the elbow will result in a complete wrist drop and inability to extend the fingers at the metacarpophalangeal joints. It should be remembered that paralysis of this nerve will not result in inability to extend the interphalangeal joints of either the thumb or digits because of the contribution to that function by the intrinsic muscles. The sensory deficit over the dorsoradial aspect of the wrist and hand resulting from radial nerve interruption is of much less significance than lesions to nerves innervating the volar side.

Various combinations of paralyses involving more than one nerve of the upper extremity are frequently encountered; those of the median and ulnar nerve are the most common. High lesions of these two nerves will produce paralyses of both the extrinsic and intrinsic muscle groups with total sensory loss over the volar aspect of the hand. More distal combined median and ulnar lesions will have their effect primarily on the intrinsic muscles, resulting in the most disabling deformities with metacarpophalangeal hyperextension, interphalangeal flexion, and thumb collapse. An inefficient pattern of digital flexion consisting of a slow distal-to-proximal, rolling grasp will result from the loss of the integrated intrinsic participation.

A number of entrapment phenomena are now recognized that may cause complete or partial paralyses, purely sensory deficits, or a combination of these alterations in any of the three major peripheral nerves of the upper extremity. Ulnar nerve compression at the elbow and median nerve compression in the carpal tunnel are among the more frequent entrapment entities.

BLOOD SUPPLY

The blood supply to the hand is carried by the radial and ulnar arteries and their branches (Fig. 1-20). The ulnar artery, which can often be palpated just lateral to the pisiform, reaches the wrist in company with the ulnar nerve immediately lateral to the flexor carpi ulnaris tendon. The artery divides at the wrist into a large branch that forms the superficial arterial arch of the hand and a smaller branch that forms the lesser part of the deep palmar arch. As it passes between the pisiform and the hamate (canal of Guyon), the ulnar artery is particularly vulnerable to repetitive trauma, which may result in thrombosis, giving rise to symptoms of vascular embarrassment and occasionally sensory abnormalities of the ulnar nerve by virtue of its close proximity to this structure.

The radial artery, which may be palpated near the proximal volar wrist crease, divides into a small superficial branch, which continues distally over the thenar eminence to complete the superficial arterial arch. The larger deep radial branch passes between the heads of the first dorsal interosseous and around the base of the thumb, where it reaches the palm to form the deep palmar arch.

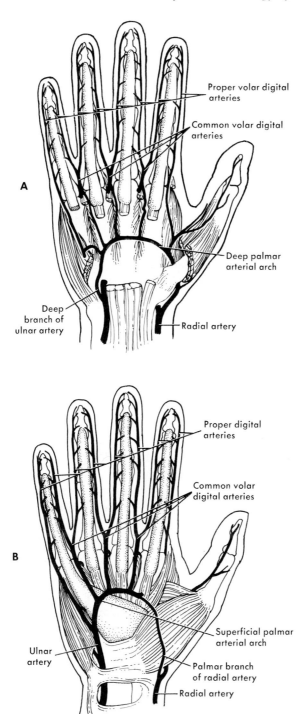

Fig. 1-20. Vascular anatomy of the hand. **A,** The deep arch is supplied by the radial artery. **B,** The superficial arch is supplied by the ulnar artery.

The superficial arterial arch gives off digital branches that bifurcate into phalangeal branches immediately below the central part of the palmar fascia. The metacarpal branches of the deep arch empty into the digital branches of the superficial arch just proximal to their bifurcation into the phalangeal arteries. It is believed by many that the superficial arterial arch is larger and more important than is the deep arch.

Although little emphasis is placed on the venous drainage of the hand, it is important to remember that the hand, like the remainder of the upper extremity, is drained by two sets of veins: a superficial group located on the superficial fascia and a deep group that travels with the arteries. The superficial venous system is the more important, and the majority of these draining vessels form a large network over the dorsum of the hand. The dorsal venous arch receives digital veins from the fingers and becomes continuous proximally with the cephalic and basilic veins on the radial and ulnar borders of the wrist. It is easy to see why injuries over the dorsum of the hand that interrupt or are prejudicial to the flow of venous drainage can result in marked congestion and edema.

SKIN AND SUBCUTANEOUS FASCIA

The palmar skin with its numerous small fibrous connections to the underlying palmar aponeurosis is a highly specialized, thickened structure with very little mobility. Numerous small blood vessels pass through the underlying subcutaneous tissues into the dermis. In contrast, the dorsal skin and subcutaneous tissue is much more loose with few anchoring fibers and a high degree of mobility. Most of the lymphatic drainage from the palmar aspect of the fingers, web areas, and hypothenar and thenar eminences flows in lymph channels on the dorsum of the hand. Clinical swelling, which frequently accompanies injury or infection, is usually a result of impaired lymph drainage.

The central, triangularly shaped palmar aponeurosis (Fig. 1-21) provides a semirigid barrier between the volar skin and the important underlying neurovascular and tendon structures. It fuses medially and laterally with the deep fascia covering the hypothenar and thenar muscles, and fasciculi extending from this thick fascial barrier extend to the proximal phalanges to fuse with the tendon sheaths on the palmar, medial, and lateral aspects. In the distal palm, septa from this palmar fascia extend to the deep transverse metacarpal ligaments forming the sides of the annular fibrous canals, allowing for the passage of the ensheathed flexor tendons and the lumbrical muscles as well as the neurovascular bundles.

Dorsally the deep fascia and extensor tendons fuse to form the roof for the dorsal subaponeurotic space, which, although not as thick as its volar counterpart, may prove restrictive to underlying fluid accumulations or intrinsic muscle swelling.

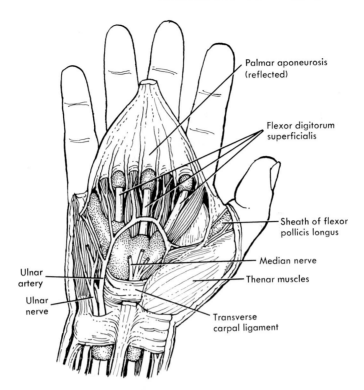

Fig. 1-21. Palmar aponeurosis reflected distally reveals septa and underlying palmar anatomy. (Modified from Lampe, E. W.: Surgical anatomy of the hand. In Clinical symposia, New York, 1969, CIBA Pharmaceutical Co., Division of CIBA-GEIGY Corp; illustrated by F. H. Netter.)

SUPERFICIAL ANATOMY

It is particularly important for the person engaged in splint preparation to thoroughly understand the surface anatomy of the forearm and hand, including the various landmarks that represent underlying anatomic structures. Respect for bony prominences and a knowledge of the position of underlying joints will be particularly important if one is to prepare splint devices that are comfortable and either immobilize or allow motion at various levels. Figs. 1-22 to 1-24 indicate the various contours of the forearm, wrist, and palm and the underlying structures that are responsible for these contours. In addition, the volar creases of the surface of the wrist and palm are depicted in relation to their underlying joint structures (Fig. 1-25) to indicate the anatomic borders that must be respected in the preparation of splints designed to allow motion at either the wrist, metacarpophalangeal, or interphalangeal joint level.

Perhaps the most vulnerable of the bony prominences of the wrist and hand are the styloid processes of the radius and ulna. By virtue of their subcutaneous

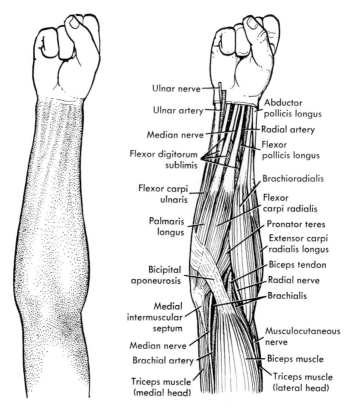

Ulnar nerve

Ulnar artery

Median nerve

Flexor digitorum sublimis

Flexor carpi ulnaris

Palmaris longus

Bicipital aponeurosis

Medial intermuscular septum

Median nerve

Brachial artery

Triceps muscle (medial head)

Abductor pollicis longus

Radial artery

Flexor pollicis longus

Brachioradialis

Flexor carpi radialis

Pronator teres

Extensor carpi radialis longus

Biceps tendon

Radial nerve

Brachialis

Musculocutaneous nerve

Biceps muscle

Triceps muscle (lateral head)

Fig. 1-22. Topographic anatomy of the volar forearm.

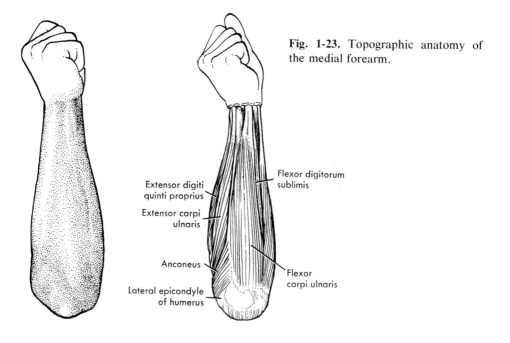

Fig. 1-23. Topographic anatomy of the medial forearm.

Extensor digiti quinti proprius

Extensor carpi ulnaris

Anconeus

Lateral epicondyle of humerus

Flexor digitorum sublimis

Flexor carpi ulnaris

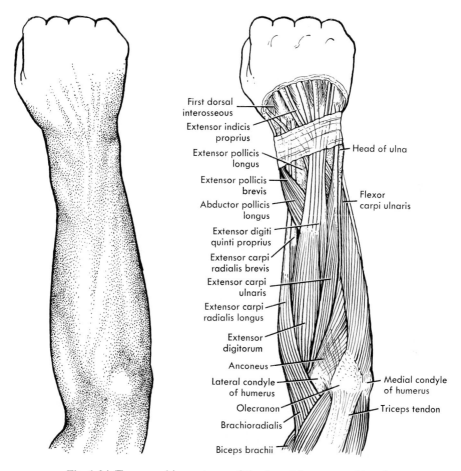

First dorsal
interosseous

Extensor indicis
proprius

Extensor pollicis
longus

Extensor pollicis
brevis

Abductor pollicis
longus

Extensor digiti
quinti proprius

Extensor carpi
radialis brevis

Extensor carpi
ulnaris

Extensor carpi
radialis longus

Extensor
digitorum

Anconeus

Lateral condyle
of humerus

Olecranon

Brachioradialis

Biceps brachii

Head of ulna

Flexor
carpi ulnaris

Medial condyle
of humerus

Triceps tendon

Fig. 1-24. Topographic anatomy of the dorsal forearm and hand.

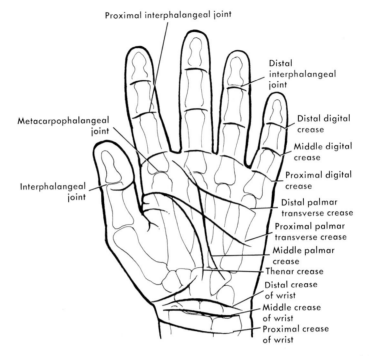

Proximal interphalangeal joint

Distal interphalangeal joint

Metacarpophalangeal joint

Distal digital crease

Middle digital crease

Proximal digital crease

Interphalangeal joint

Distal palmar transverse crease

Proximal palmar transverse crease

Middle palmar crease

Thenar crease

Distal crease of wrist

Middle crease of wrist

Proximal crease of wrist

Fig. 1-25. Relationship of the volar skin creases to the underlying wrist and digital joints. Metacarpophalangeal joints lie at the level of the distal palmar crease.

position, these areas are particularly vulnerable to poorly contoured splints. Great care must be taken to avoid appliances that place unequal pressure against these osseous structures.

FUNCTIONAL PATTERNS

The prehensile function of the hand is dependent on the integrity of the kinetic chain of bones and joints extending from the wrist to the distal phalanges. Interruptions of the transverse and longitudinal arch systems formed by these structures will always result in instability, deformity, or functional loss at a more proximal or distal level. Similarly, the balanced synergism-antagonism relationship between the long extrinsic muscles and the intrinsic muscles is a requisite for the composite functions required for both power and precision functions of the hand. It is important to recognize that the hand cannot function well without normal sensory input from all areas.

Many attempts have been made to classify the different patterns of hand function, and various types of grasp and pinch have been described. Perhaps the more simplified analysis of power grasp and precision handling as proposed by Napier (1968) and refined by Flatt (1972) is the easiest to consider.

As generally stated, power grip is a combination of strong thumb motion with the powerful flexion of the ring and small fingers on the ulnar side of the hand. The

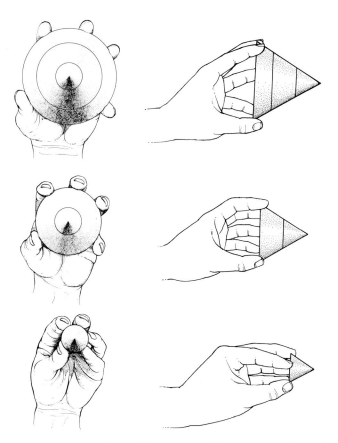

Fig. 1-26. Progressive alterations in precision grasp with changes in object size. Adaptation takes place primarily at the carpometacarpal joint of the thumb and the metacarpophalangeal joints of the digits.

radial half of the hand employing the delicate tripod of pinch between the thumb, index, and long fingers is responsible for more delicate precision function.

An analysis of hand functions requires that one consider the thumb and the remainder of the hand as two separate parts. Rotation of the thumb into an opposing position is a requirement of almost any hand function, whether it be strong grasp or delicate pinch. The wide range of motion permitted at the carpometacarpal joint is extremely important in allowing the thumb to be correctly positioned. Stability at this joint is a requirement of almost all prehensile activities and is ensured by a unique ligamentous arrangement, which allows mobility in the midposition and provides stability at the extremes. As can be seen in Fig. 1-26, the thumb moves through a wide arc from the side of the index finger tip to the tip of the small finger, and the adaptation that occurs between the thumb and digits as progressively smaller objects are held occurs primarily at the metacarpophalangeal joints of the digits and the carpometacarpal joint of the thumb.

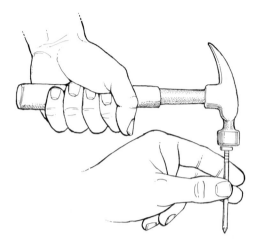

Fig. 1-27. Strong power grip imparted primarily by the thumb, ring, and small fingers around the hammer handle with delicate precision tip grip employed to hold the nail.

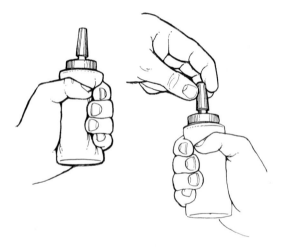

Fig. 1-28. Power grip used to hold the squeeze bottle with precision handling of the bottle top by the opposite hand.

For power grip the wrist is in an extended position that allows the extrinsic digital flexors to press the object firmly against the palm while the thumb is closed tightly around the object. The thumb, ring, and small fingers are the most important participants in this strong grasp function, and the importance of the ulnar border digits cannot be minimized (Fig. 1-27).

In precision grasp, wrist position is less important, and the thumb is opposed to the semiflexed fingers with the intrinsic tendons providing most of the finger movement. Certain activities may require combinations of power and precision grasp as seen in Fig. 1-28. Pinching between the thumb and the combined index

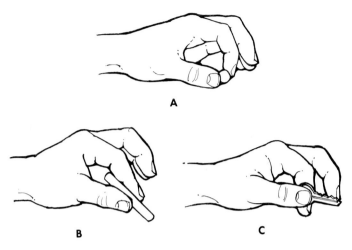

Fig. 1-29. Types of precision grip. **A,** Tip grip. **B,** Palmar grip. **C,** Lateral grip. (Modified from Flatt, A. E.: The care of the rheumatoid hand, ed. 3, St. Louis, 1974, The C. V. Mosby Co.)

and long fingers is a further refinement of precision grip and may be classified as either tip grip, lateral grip, or palmar grip (Fig. 1-29), depending on the portions of the phalanges brought to bear on the object being handled. In these functions the strong contracture of the adductor pollicis brings the thumb into contact against the tip or sides of the index or index and long fingers with digital resistance imparted by the first and second dorsal interossei. The size of the object being handled will dictate whether large thumb and digital surfaces, as in palmar grip, or smaller surfaces, as in lateral or tip grasp, are utilized. Flatt (1974) has pointed out that the dual importance of rotation and flexion of the thumb is often ignored in the preparation of splints, which permit only tip grip because the thumb cannot oppose the pulp of the fingers to produce palmar grip.

The patterns of action of the normal hand depend on the mobility of the skeletal arches and alterations of the configuration of these arches is produced by the balanced function of the extrinsic and intrinsic muscles. Whereas the extrinsic contribution resulting from the large powerful forearm muscle groups is more important to hand strength, the fine precision action imparted by the intrinsic musculature gives the hand an enormous variety of capabilities. Although one need not specifically memorize the various patterns of pinch, grasp, and combined hand functions, it is important to understand the underlying contribution of the various muscle-tendon groups, both extrinsic and intrinsic, to these activities. Injuries or diseases that affect the integrity of the arch system or disrupt or paralyze the extrinsic or intrinsic muscles will have a profound impact on hand function.

It is hoped that this chapter will serve as a reference guide for the important anatomic and kinesiologic considerations presented in the ensuing chapters on hand splinting.

CHAPTER 2

Classification and nomenclature of splints and splint components

Because hand splinting encompasses a profusion of devices and terminology, and because similar splints may be used for dissimilar purposes, description and classification of various splints is often fraught with confusion, redundancy, and omission. Historically, there has been a variety of splint classifications, including groupings according to purpose, configuration, mechanical properties, power source, material, and anatomic site. Each method has advantages and disadvantages, and, although some classification systems are more precise than others, none effectively provides a clear description and separation of individual splints and components. The need for common descriptive splint terminology has been apparent to clinicians, students, and patients for years.

The purpose of this chapter is threefold: (1) to familiarize the reader with basic historical concepts that comprise the foundation of current splinting techniques by reviewing six established methods of splint classification; (2) to introduce a new method of splint classification based on force complexity, joints involved, and kinematic purpose; and (3) to provide a common vocabulary of splint component terminology to facilitate further discussion and communication.

ESTABLISHED SPLINT CLASSIFICATIONS

Despite discrepancies, familiarity with the various methods of splint categorization provides a basis for understanding the origins of current hand splinting methods and general splinting nomenclature. As has been noted, splints may be classified according to the intent or purpose of application.

Purpose of application

Splints may be designed to *prevent deformity* by substituting for weak or absent muscle strength as in peripheral nerve injuries, spinal cord injuries, and neuromuscular diseases. They may be used to *support, protect, or immobilize joints,* allowing healing to occur after tendon, vascular, nerve, joint, or soft tissue injury or inflammation. *Correction of existing deformity* represents another commonly encountered reason for splint application. To achieve the full potential of active joint motion of the hand, the stretching of joint and tendon adhesions will often require the prolonged slow, gentle, passive traction that can best be provided by splinting. Splints also may provide directional *control* for coordination problems and serve as a basis for the *attachment* of specialized devices that may facilitate and enhance hand function.

External configuration

External configuration has often served as a basis for the categorization of hand splints. This method includes the subcategorization of bar splints, spring splints, contoured splints, and combinations thereof.

Bar splints. Bar splints, because of the narrowness of design, must be fabricated in strong inelastic materials such as stainless steel, aluminum, and the thicker high-temperature plastics. There are two major forms of bar splints (Fig. 2-1) from which most other splints derive their design concepts.

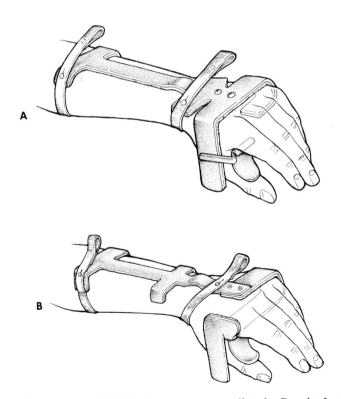

Fig. 2-1. Bar splints are exemplified by long opponens splints by Rancho Los Amigos (**A**) and Bennett (Warm Springs) (**B**) differ in placement of the uninterrupted metacarpal bar.

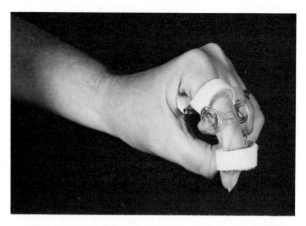

Fig. 2-2. The Capner splint provides dynamic extension assist to the proximal interphalangeal joint through forces generated by bilateral springs and a three-point pressure system.

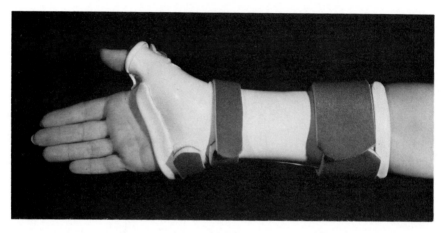

Fig. 2-3. Contoured splints are often more comfortable to wear because of increased surface contact with the extremity.

Spring splints. Spring splints, as exemplified by many of the Bunnell, Capner, and Wynn Parry splints, rely on three-point pressure and spring-action forces to provide dynamic mobilization (Fig. 2-2).

Contoured splints. Because of their ease of fabrication with low-temperature materials that may be fitted directly to the patients, contoured splints have revolutionized hand splinting techniques, moving them out of the realm of the orthotist and into therapy clinics and physician's offices (Fig. 2-3). Since the low-temperature materials lack the rigidity required, splint designs of necessity have become wider. This has fortuitously resulted in greater patient comfort because of decreased splint pressure from an increased area of force application.

Combinations. Combinations of bar, spring, and contoured splints comprise the fourth subcategory. Engen, Bailor, and the Wire-foam splints (Fig. 2-4) are examples of how the strength of metal may be coalesced with the close-fitting capabilities of plastics.

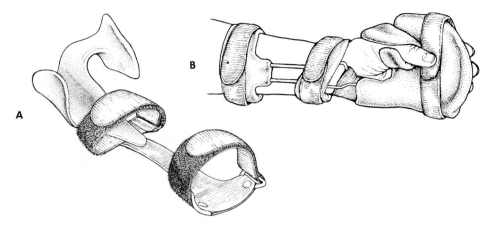

Fig. 2-4. The Engen (**A**) and Wire-foam (**B**) splints combine metal and plastic to produce a durable, close-fitting, adjustable splint.

Mechanical characteristics

Hand splints may also be grouped according to inherent mechanical characteristics, resulting in two major subdivisions: static splints and dynamic splints. *Static splints* have no moving parts and are used to provide support and immobilization, whereas *dynamic splints* employ traction devices such as rubber bands, springs, cords, or Velcro strips to alter the range of passive motion of a joint or joints. Confusion arises with this method of classification, since some splints possess static properties but function dynamically by means of consecutive configuration alterations as exemplified by cylinder casts and thumb web spacers.

Source of power

The source of power is another categoric method that divides dynamic splints into those which utilize internal power and those which provide external power. These splints are often more complicated to fabricate than are some of the more temporary splints, requiring durable materials, mechanical joints, and tension-adjusting systems. These are frequently used in cases of severe upper extremity paralysis. Dynamic *internally powered splints* rely on the use of the patient's residual muscle power at a given joint to produce motion of nonfunctional joints following various paralytic conditions (Fig. 2-5). Dynamic *externally powered splints* are driven by an external source such as a battery or carbon dioxide artificial muscle. Generally, both the internal and external power splints permit gross grasp through wrist extension, or tenodesis effect.

Materials

A fifth means of classification is based on the materials from which splints are fabricated. Categoric divisions include *metal, plaster, and plastic;* subcategories within this classification system change as technologic advances occur.

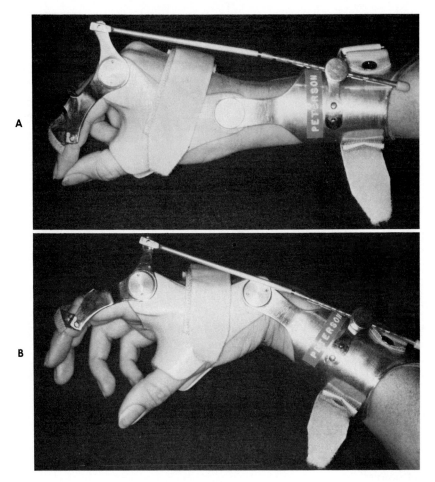

Fig. 2-5. Digital grasp and release patterns are controlled by active wrist extension (**A**) and gravity-assisted flexion (**B**) in this tenodesis splint.

Anatomic part

The final classification system relates to the anatomic part splinted, as in *wrist splints, finger splints, or thumb splints*. These subcategories are grouped according to the primary intent of a given splint but do not describe the existence of secondary joints that may also be affected by the splint.

•   •   •

This retrospective consideration of splint classification techniques is important because it encompasses a cumulative framework of splinting knowledge. In studying newer splinting techniques it must be recognized that pathologic conditions of the hand have not been altered, neither have the principles of mechanics, design, construction, and fit. Only the materials have changed, permitting modern clinicians to use splint components that are similar in function to those used by their predecessors but which are more easily contoured and fabricated.

DESCRIPTIVE CLASSIFICATION SYSTEM

The intent of introducing a new method of splint classification is to provide a more definitive means of grouping splints based on three criteria: (1) the types of splinting forces employed and the spatial planes in which they occur, (2) the anatomic site of emphasis, and (3) the primary kinematic goal of the splint. When describing a given splint, one uses three adjectives to delineate the "how," "where," and "why" of the splint, resulting in such descriptive phases as "complex wrist extension splint," "compound finger flexion splint," or "simple proximal interphalangeal (PIP) immobilization splint."

How?

The first category, or the "how" of a splint, is divided into three subcategories that allow grouping according to the complexity of the splinting forces and the planes in which they affect motion. To control articular motion, a *simple splint* affects motion at a single or multiple joints within a segment in a similar manner (Fig. 2-6). To control articular motion, a *compound splint* affects motion at two or more joints within a segment in a dissimilar manner (Fig. 2-7). Complex splints are those designed to influence the impact of the amplitude of the long extrinsic tendons on a given joint or joints. By incorporating the wrist in a splint acting on the digits it is possible to negate the extrinsic muscle forces (Fig. 2-8). Similarly, two-level complex splints may be utilized to improve motion at the wrist by immobilizing the digits in a favorable position.

Where?

The anatomic site of emphasis defines the "where" of the splint. If all joints of a digital ray are similarly affected, the term "finger" or "thumb" is applied.

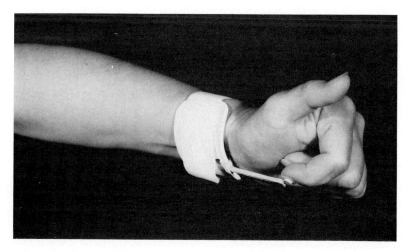

Fig. 2-6. A simple finger flexion splint exerts a similar force on all joints of the digit.

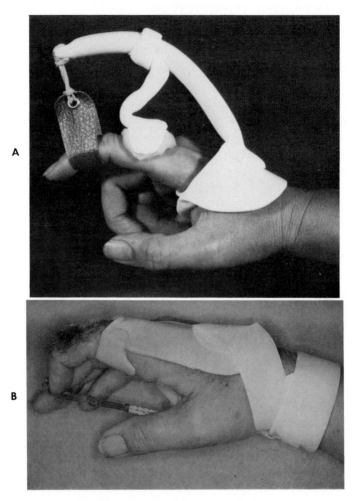

Fig. 2-7. These compound proximal interphalangeal joint extension (**A**) and flexion (**B**) splints differ in force direction but mechanically function alike.

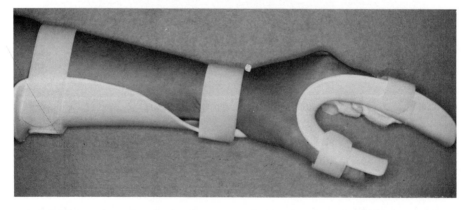

Fig. 2-8. The resting pan splint is an example of a complex finger immobilization splint.

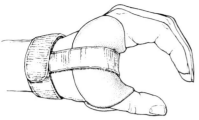

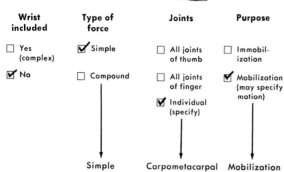

Fig. 2-9. This graphic interpretation of the descriptive splint classification method illustrates the fundamental concepts involved. **A,** Simple carpometacarpal (CMC) mobilization splint. **B,** Complex compound thumb and PIP extension splint.

A

Wrist included	Type of force	Joints	Purpose
☐ Yes (complex)	☑ Simple	☐ All joints of thumb	☐ Immobilization
☑ No	☐ Compound	☐ All joints of finger	☑ Mobilization (may specify motion)
		☑ Individual (specify)	
↓	↓	↓	↓
Simple		Carpometacarpal	Mobilization

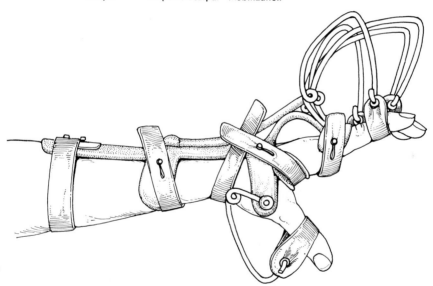

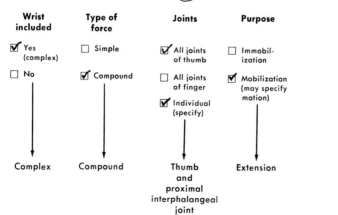

B

Wrist included	Type of force	Joints	Purpose
☑ Yes (complex)	☐ Simple	☑ All joints of thumb	☐ Immobilization
☐ No	☑ Compound	☐ All joints of finger	☑ Mobilization (may specify motion)
		☑ Individual (specify)	
↓	↓	↓	↓
Complex	Compound	Thumb and proximal interphalangeal joint	Extension

If, however, the emphasis of the splint is more specific, the individual joint level(s) involved should be named. For example, a splint affecting both the proximal inter-phalangeal (PIP) and distal interphalangeal (DIP) joints would be labeled inter-phalangeal (IP), whereas one whose forces are directed to the PIP joint alone would be referred to specifically as PIP.

Why?

The third and final adjective refers to the "why" of the splint and is defined by kinematic terminology. What is the intent of the splint? Does if flex, rotate, or abduct, or is its primary purpose to immobilize? The addition of this functional purpose completes the descriptive triad and provides an immediate visualization of a given splint type.

Combining of the three adjectives results in a descriptive splint classification based on well-defined categories that are large enough to include an array of splints but small enough to clearly delineate specific force, site, and purpose characteristics (Fig. 2-9).

SPLINT COMPONENT TERMINOLOGY

A splint is no more than a series of specialized parts that perform specific functions. Some of these parts directly affect the position of the hand, whereas others maintain the alignment and spatial interrelationships between the various splint components. When assessing a hand with the intent of applying a splint, one should not think of the splint as a whole, but rather as interconnected parts, each meeting a specific need for a given clinical hand problem. There are no routine splints that can be prescribed for a given pathologic situation. No one has decreed that similarly functioning splint parts must look alike or can be used only with certain diagnoses. Each patient presents different problems, even though the specific injury or disease may be similar to those of others. The patient must be approached without preconceived ideas, allowing for the creation of a splint, part by part, that meets not only physical but emotional and environmental requirements. An inability to accommodate to these individual factors is the main cause for failure of many commercial splints. Remember, patients and their hands do not come in small, medium, and large!

To effectively accomplish component splint designing, a sound knowledge of the basic splint parts and their purposes is essential. As was noted earlier in this chapter, each splint part has a task for which it has been designed. It may vary in shape from splint to splint, but its purpose will remain constant. Some parts mobilize, some support, others stabilize, and still others provide attachment sites. Following is an alphabetic listing of splint parts, their purposes, and pertinent information concerning each component. This list is meant to provide a basic foundation of common language for further communication. It should not be viewed as definitive, but rather should be added to, elaborated on, and deleted from as the splint maker accumulates experience and expertise.

C bar (Fig. 2-10)

This bar is fitted in the first web space for the purpose of maintaining or increasing the distance between the first and second metacarpal bones. The C bar is frequently elongated to incorporate a thumb post or an index proximal phalanx support. Its width should not impede the movement of the mobile fourth and fifth metacarpals. Care should be taken to maintain through exercise full metacarpophalangeal (MP) flexion of the index finger when a C bar is used with an index phalangeal extension.

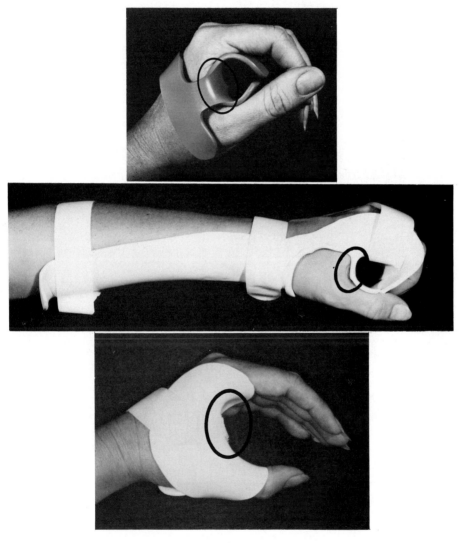

Fig. 2-10. Although dissimilar in appearance, all three of these splints employ C bars to maintain the first web space.

Connector bar (Fig. 2-11)

This piece of splinting material maintains the alignment and position of individual splint parts. Depending on specific location and purpose in regard to the overall splint design, connector bars may or may not be constructed of materials homologous to the splint.

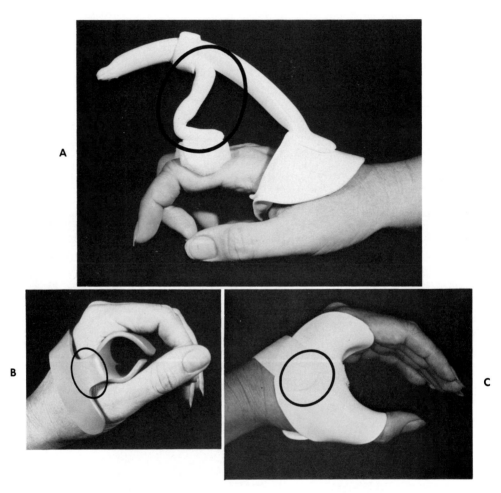

Fig. 2-11. A connector bar may be a separate piece (**A** and **B**), or it may be integrated into the body of the splint (**C**).

Crossbar (Fig. 2-12)

This transverse medial or lateral extension, in combination with similar bars, provides rigid splint stability on the forearm and hand. Crossbars may be used in pairs, singly in three-point configuration with the most distal point often serving as a wrist deviation bar, or, in the case of a highly contoured splint, with the proximal and distal bars molded together bilaterally to form the continuous lateral aspects of a forearm trough.

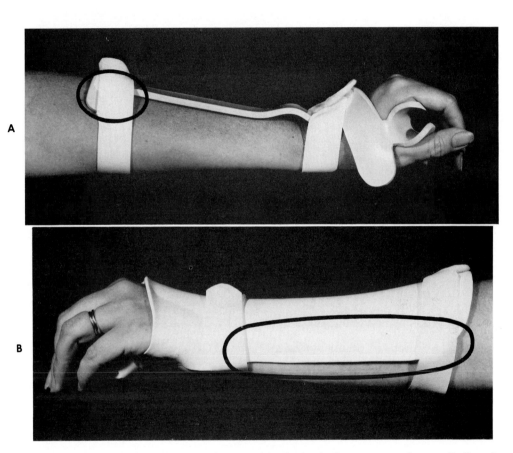

Fig. 2-12. A, Extrinsic crossbars often provide the basis for strap attachment. **B,** Fused crossbars increase splint strength.

Cuff or strap (Fig. 2-13)

This splint attachment is usually of a softer, more pliable material that holds the splint in place on the extremity. Cuffs are frequently wider than straps and disperse pressure over half the lateral width of the segment in addition to increasing the area of force application on the dorsal or volar surface, resulting in greater patient comfort (see also discussion of finger cuff).

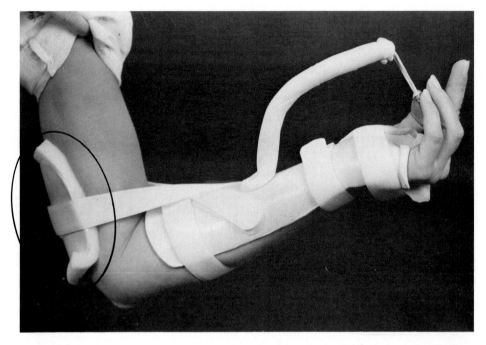

Fig. 2-13. A triceps cuff prevents distal migration of this complex metacarpophalangeal flexion splint.

Deviation bar (Fig. 2-14)

A deviation bar is any static component that positions the wrist or fingers on a coronal plane. To be fully effective, the height of this ulnar or radial bar should be no less than half the thickness of the segment to which it is fitted and no greater than the full segment thickness. These bars are almost always continuations of the splint itself, providing contoured strength in addition to positioning.

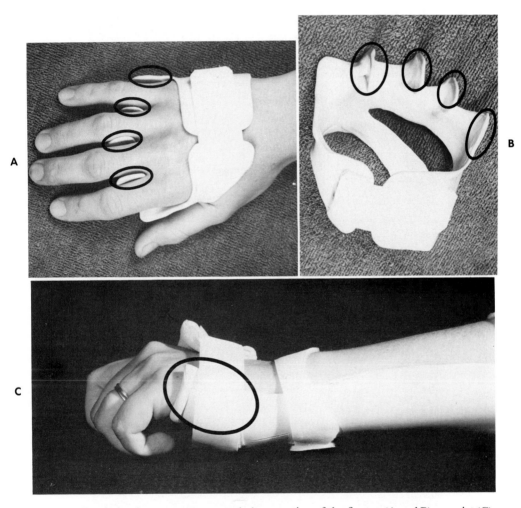

Fig. 2-14. Deviation bars prevent coronal plane motion of the fingers (**A** and **B**) or wrist (**C**). (**A** and **B** courtesy K. P. MacBain, O.T.R., Vancouver, British Columbia.)

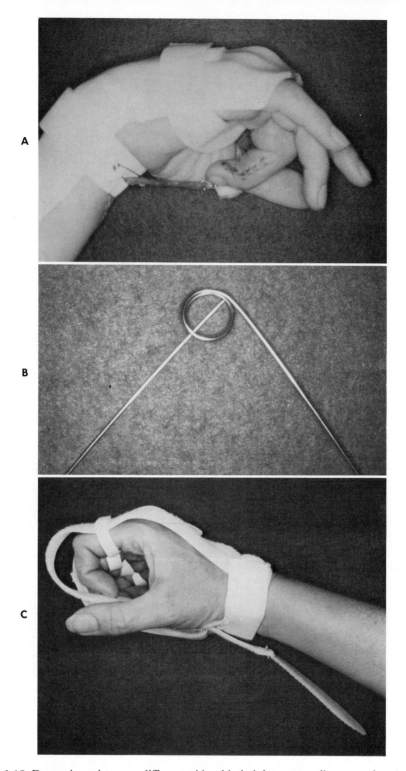

Fig. 2-15. Dynamic assists may differ considerably in inherent tensile properties. **A,** Rubber band. **B,** Spring wire. **C,** Velcro strap.

Dynamic assist or traction device (Fig. 2-15)

This splint part creates a mobilizing force on a segment, resulting in passive or passive-assistive motion of a joint or successive joints. Dynamic traction devices may be made of self-adjusting resiliant or elastic materials such as rubber or spring wire, or they may consist of less tensile materials such as Velcro, cording, or leather that rely on the wearer for adjustment.

Finger cuff (Fig. 2-16)

This splint component circumferentially attaches a dynamic assist to the finger. Finger cuffs are most often made of a flexible but inelastic material; in the case of extension traction, they must be cut to allow full flexion of proximal and distal finger joints.

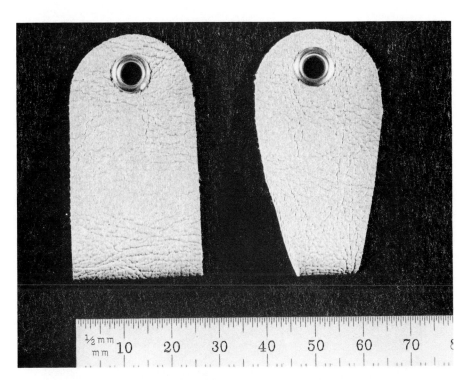

Fig. 2-16. Trimmed finger cuffs should not impede digital flexion.

Fingernail attachment (Fig. 2-17)

A fingernail attachment is any device or material that, when fastened to the fingernail, provides an attachment site for a dynamic assist or traction. It may be adhered to the nail with fast-setting ethyl cyanoacrylate glue or, in the case of a loop, sutured through the distal free edge of the nail body.

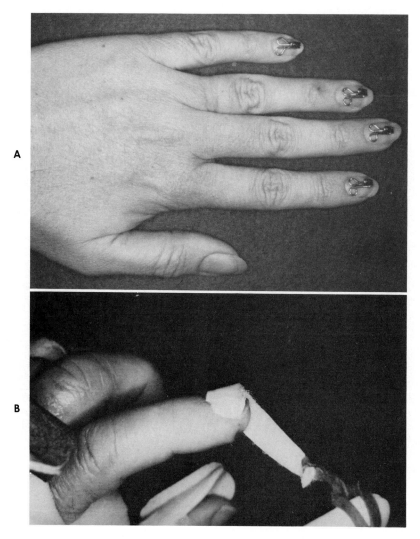

Fig. 2-17. Frequently used fingernail attachment devices. **A,** Dress hooks. **B,** Velcro hook tabs.

Forearm bar or trough (Fig. 2-18)

This longitudinal splint part rests proximal to the wrist on one or more surfaces of the forearm. This bar statically provides the leverage to support the weight of the hand and should be at least two thirds the length of the forearm to minimize resultant pressure.

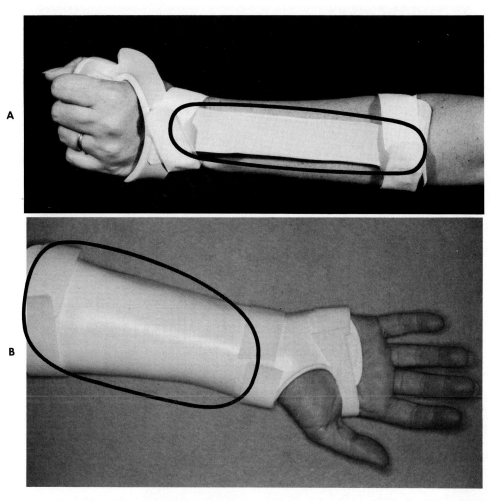

Fig. 2-18. A forearm bar (**A**) or trough (**B**) must be long enough to comfortably support the proximally transferred weight of the hand.

Hypothenar bar (Fig. 2-19)

The bar that palmarly supports the ulnar aspect of the transverse metacarpal arch is called a hypothenar bar and is frequently the continuation of a dorsal or volar metacarpal bar. It should not inhibit flexion of the ring and small metacarpophalangeal joints.

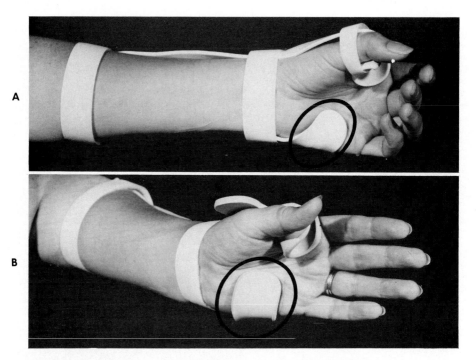

Fig. 2-19. A hypothenar bar supports the fourth and fifth metacarpals.

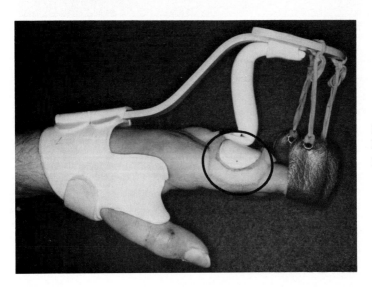

Fig. 2-20. For legend see opposite page.

Joint

The mechanical overlapping of splint components results in either an axis of rotation (one rivet) or a solid immobile bond (provided by two or more rivets or by a cohesion of homologous material surfaces).

Lumbrical bar (Fig. 2-20)

This bar extends over the dorsal aspect of one or more proximal phalanges and prevents a predetermined amount of metacarpophalangeal extension or hyperextension. In the case of multiple fingers, the lumbrical bar also maintains

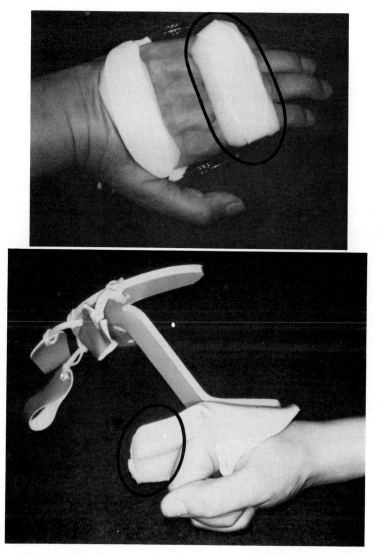

Fig. 2-20. Although dissimilar in appearance, these lumbrical bars all control the degree of metacarpophalangeal extension.

the transverse arch at the phalangeal level. Because of the fragility of the dorsal skin and the magnified forces of a dynamic splint, padding is often required for pressure dissemination. The radial and ulnar sides of a lumbrical bar should curve volarly to half the width of the proximal phalanx to prevent lateral displacement of the finger or fingers from under the bar. Longitudinally a lumbrical bar should extend a minimum of two thirds the length of the proximal phalanx.

Metacarpal bar (Fig. 2-21)

This type of bar supports the transverse metacarpal arch dorsally or volarly. A correctly fitted metacarpal bar should allow full motion of the second through fifth metacarpophalangeal joints. The ulnar and radial extensions of a metacarpal bar frequently include a hypothenar bar or an opponens bar, respectively.

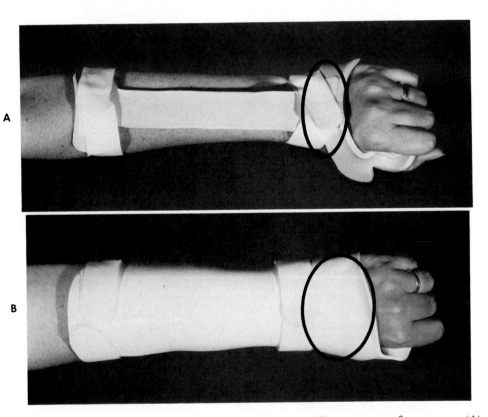

Fig. 2-21. Longitudinal measurements of dorsal metacarpal bars may vary from narrow (**A**) to those which incorporate or nearly incorporate the full length of the metacarpal(s) (**B**).

Opponens bar (Fig. 2-22)

This component, usually in conjunction with a C bar, positions the first metacarpal in various degrees of abduction and opposition while preventing radiodorsal motion of the first metacarpal.

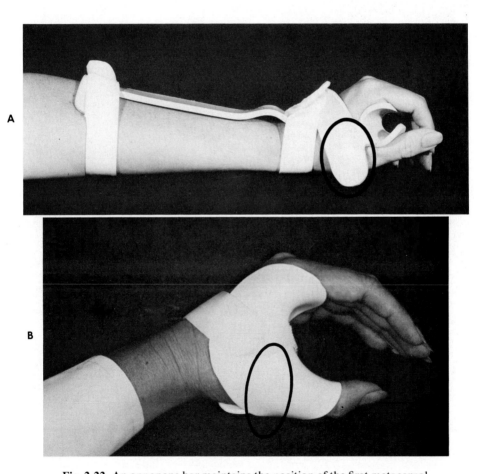

Fig. 2-22. An opponens bar maintains the position of the first metacarpal.

Outrigger (Fig. 2-23)

   This splint part is extended out from the main body of the splint for the purpose of positioning dynamic assists or traction devices. To maintain correct alignment of the traction devices, the length of an outrigger must be adjusted as change occurs in passive range of motion of the joint(s) being mobilized. Because the magnitude of the dynamic traction will be lessened with instability of its proximal attachment, an outrigger should furnish a rigid or near-rigid foundation for force propagation.

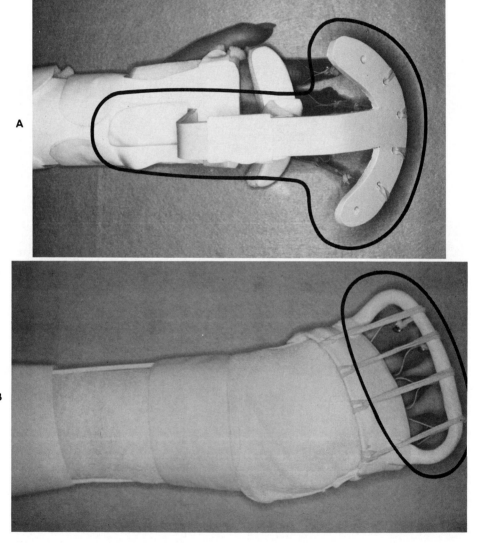

Fig. 2-23. For legend see opposite page.

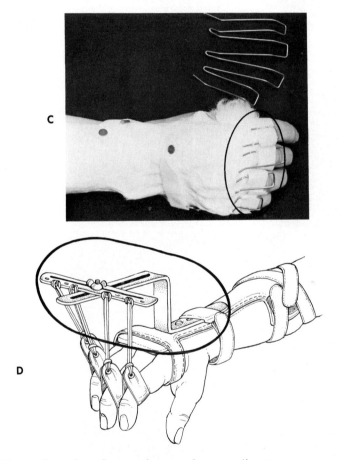

Fig. 2-23. The configuration of an outrigger varies according to purpose and construction material. (C from Hollis, I.: Innovative splinting ideas. In Hunter, J. M., et al., editors: Rehabilitation of the hand, St. Louis, 1978, The C. V. Mosby Co.)

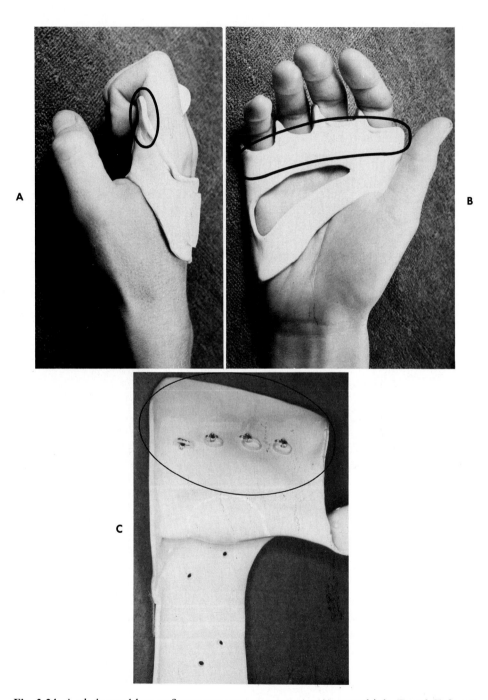

Fig. 2-24. A phalangeal bar or finger pan may support one (**A**) or multiple (**B** and **C**) finger segments. (**A** and **B** courtesy K. P. MacBain, O.T.R., Vancouver, British Columbia.)

Phalangeal bar or finger pan (Fig. 2-24)

The finger pan or phalangeal bar maintains the transverse and longitudinal arches distally when multiple rays or segments are involved, while providing dorsal or volar support to the phalanges. If the phalangeal bar immobilizes only a portion of a segment, care should be taken not to inhibit the motion of adjacent joints. The medial and lateral continuations of this bar frequently end in deviation bars, providing coronal plane control and splint durability through contour.

Prop (Fig. 2-25)

A prop is an attachment that places the splinted extremity away from a supporting surface to prevent pressure from prolonged gravitational force.

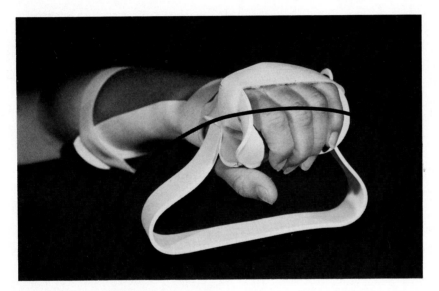

Fig. 2-25. A prop may be of assistance in preventing pressure breakdown in severe upper extremity paralysis.

Reinforcement bar (Fig. 2-26)

This adjunctive splint component increases the strength and durability of the splint. The zealous use of reinforcement bars is frequently indicative of poor splint design or material choice. Contoured material and the incorporation of sound mechanical principles is far more effective in providing splint strength than is the retrospective trussing with layers of material.

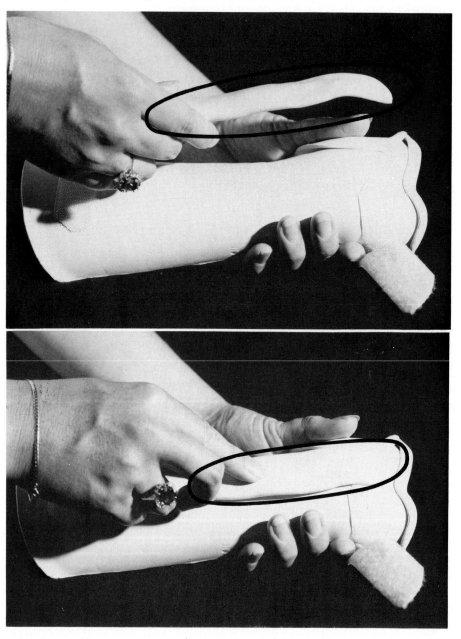

Fig. 2-26. A contoured reinforcement bar may be used to provide additional strength to a splint.

Thumb post (Fig. 2-27)

This device statically supports the proximal and distal phalanges of the thumb and is usually a distal extension of a C bar. When only the proximal phalanx is immobilized, full interphalangeal joint motion should not be inhibited by overextension of the thumb post distally. Since the configuration of this bar is often long and narrow, contouring of the material to half of the thickness of the splinted segment will allow for increased stability. When the immobile thumb is to be used in functional activities, it is preferable to design the thumb post to fit dorsally, allowing the gripping surfaces of the thumb to have sensory reception.

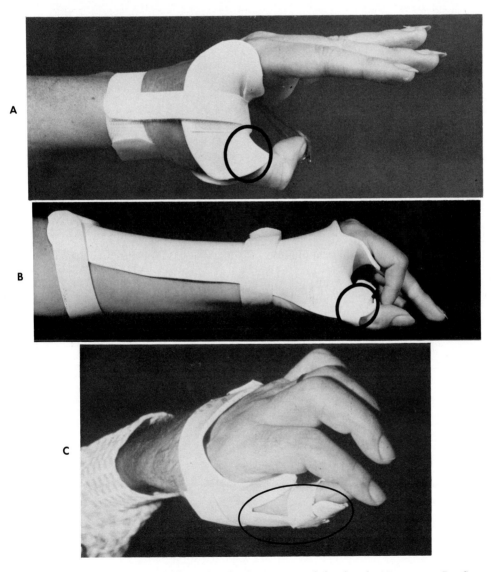

A

B

C

Fig. 2-27. A thumb post positions the distal segments of the thumb. (C courtesy Pat Samuels, O.T.R., Indianapolis, Indiana.)

Wrist bar (Fig. 2-28)

Any splint part that supports the carpal area of the extremity is a wrist bar. This bar frequently connects to the forearm bar proximally and the metacarpal bar distally. The positional attitude of this bar in the sagittal plane exerts substantial influence on the kinetic interrelationships among anatomic structures; as a result, the wrist bar must be positioned advantageously and with deliberation.

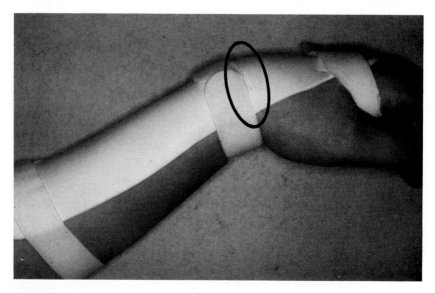

Fig. 2-28. A wrist bar placed in flexion will augment extrinsic finger extension.

SUMMARY

Although one must be cognizant of the various classification systems that have been offered for hand splints, it is important to avoid the confusion that will result from the redundancy of these systems. More important, the clinician involved in splint preparation should have a thorough knowledge of the nomenclature of the entire spectrum of splint parts, their capabilities, and indications. A creative flexibility must be developed that allows the experienced splint maker to draw from a large assortment of splint components in the preparation of a splint that will best suit the requirements of a particular hand problem. Adherence to a limited classification system may narrow these fabrication options and fail to adequately respond to the almost unlimited assortment of individual situations that exist in the diseased or injured hand. This chapter introduces a classification system that integrates force complexity, joints influenced, and kinematic purpose in an effort to provide a simple splint description terminology. We hope that this type of approach will best allow for a more accurate description of a given splint, thereby aiding therapists and physicians in the difficult area of communication.

CHAPTER 3

Mechanical principles

Reduce pressure by increasing the area of force application.

Control parallel force systems by increasing the mechanical advantage.

Use optimum rotational force when mobilizing a joint by dynamic traction.

Consider the torque effect on a joint.

Consider the relative degree of passive mobility of successive joints within the longitudinal segmental kinetic chain.

Consider the effects of reciprocal parallel forces when designing splints and placing straps.

Increase material strength by providing contour.

Eliminate friction.

Because splinting consists of the external application of forces to the extremity, understanding of the basic mechanical principles involved is an essential prerequisite to the design, construction, and fitting of all hand splints. Many therapists have learned through trial and error the basic concepts of mechanics, deductively choosing an approach that yields the most favorable result. Few, however, have the opportunity, expertise, or time to specifically analyze the differences among the available methods. Physicians, although usually possessing a more formal understanding of biomechanics, frequently do not apply this knowledge to splinting in clinical situations, accepting without question a poorly functioning splint that will ultimately produce less favorable results.

The purpose of this chapter is to integrate material from the field of mechanical engineering with the fundamental knowledge of the medical specialist as it pertains to splinting. To clarify the mechanical concepts involved, scale diagrams, red force arrows, and simple formulas illustrate the basic principles. For a more in-depth explanation, additional mathematic equations are presented in Appendix A. Gravitational forces have not been included in the examples in this chapter so that the specific principles may be emphasized and further clarified.

PRINCIPLES

Increase the area of force application. Because splinting materials are various forms of solid substances, their improper application to the extremity may cause damage to the cutaneous surface and underlying soft tissue as a result of excessive pressure. This often occurs in areas in which there is minimal subcutaneous tissue to disperse pressure such as over bony prominences or in areas where the inherent structure of the splint predisposes to increased pressure because of mechanical counterforces.

The formula

$$\text{Pressure} = \frac{\text{Total force}}{\text{Area of force application}}$$

indicates that a force of 25 grams applied over an area of 1 cm by 1 cm would result in a pressure of 0.25 gram per square millimeter. If, however, the same 25 grams of force were distributed over an area of 5 cm by 5 cm, the pressure per square millimeter would be decreased to 0.01 gram, or $\frac{1}{25}$ the pressure per square millimeter. In other words, increasing the area of force application will decrease the pressure.

Clinically this has the following implications: (1) wider, longer splints are more comfortable than short, narrow splints (Fig. 3-1); (2) rolled edges on the proximal and distal aspect of a volar splint and the distal aspect of a dorsal splint cause less pressure than do straight edges (Fig. 3-2); (3) continuous uniform pressure over a bony prominence is preferable to unequal pressure on the prominence (Fig. 3-3); and (4) because some splint components must be narrow and the resultant force great, a contiguous fit is paramount (Fig. 3-4). Generally, a continuous force applied to the extremity should not exceed 50 grams per square centimeter.

Padded materials such as heavy felt or foam rubber give uniform pressure

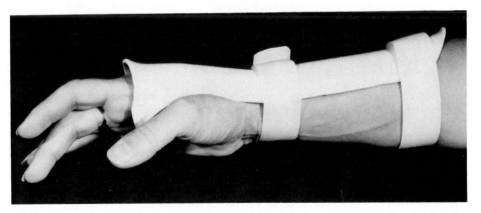

Fig. 3-1. Because of minimized pressure forces and improved mechanical factors, patient comfort is enhanced by splints with greater contact area.

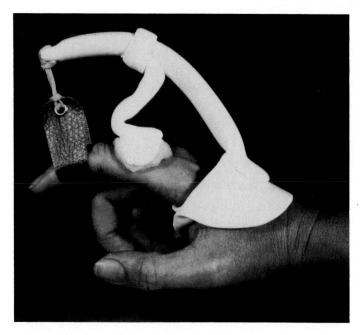

Fig. 3-2. Rolled edges allow for dissemination of pressure over a greater area, as illustrated in the C bar of this splint.

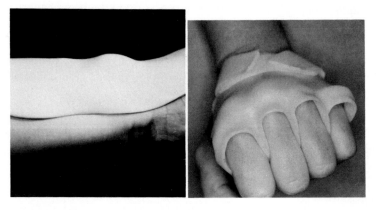

Fig. 3-3. A congruous fit over bony prominences will reduce the possibility of soft tissue damage by evenly dispersing pressure forces over a larger area.

distribution because of their inherent properties and are valuable in reducing pressure in areas in which the forces are great and the splint is narrow. Padding may be appropriate in such instances, but the zealous use of padding should not substitute for care in designing, fabricating, and fitting the splint.

Using an increased area of application to disperse the forces causing pressure is also important in the construction of a splint. Rounded internal corners diminish

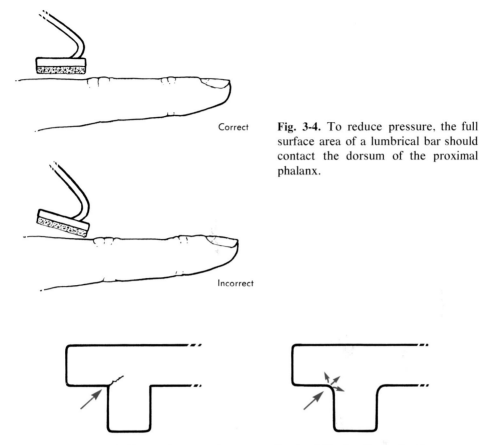

Correct

Incorrect

Fig. 3-4. To reduce pressure, the full surface area of a lumbrical bar should contact the dorsum of the proximal phalanx.

Fig. 3-5. Rounded internal corners increase splint durability by dissipating forces.

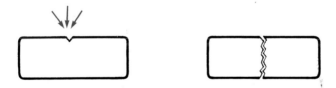

Fig. 3-6. An edge imperfection creates force convergence and increases the chances for material fracture.

the effects of force on the splint material (Fig. 3-5), as do continuously smooth edges (Fig. 3-6). In addition, rounded external corners and edges decrease the possibility of excessive pressure on underlying skin.

   Increase the mechanical advantage. The design and construction of splints should be adapted to include use of favorable force systems. Many splints fail because of patient discomfort or because of fractured components. These problems may result from inattention to the lever systems at play between the splint and the extremity or between the individual splint parts.

If the splinted forearm, wrist, and hand are viewed as a parallel force system with the wrist being the axis (A), the hand being the weight or resistance (R), and the forearm providing the counterforce to the force (F) of the proximal end of the forearm trough of the splint, the splint itself may be considered a first-class lever (Fig. 3-7) and may be further analyzed as to force lines of action, moment arms, and resultant forces. With the wrist in neutral, the forearm trough works as a force arm (FA), the perpendicular distance between the axis and the force line of action (FLA). The volar metacarpal bar functions as the resistance arm (RA), the perpendicular distance between the axis and resistance line of action (RLA) (Fig.

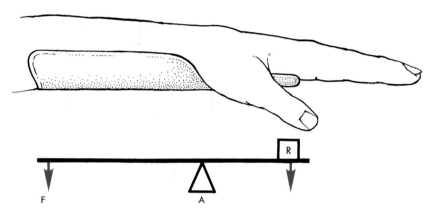

Fig. 3-7. Many splints may be functionally classified as first-class levers. *F*, Force; *A*, axis; *R*, resistance.

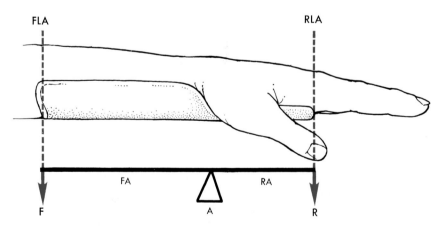

Fig. 3-8. Identification of mechanical terminology as it relates to a first-class lever system expedites subsequent force analysis. *FLA*, Force line of action; *FA*, force arm (perpendicular between axis and FLA); *A*, axis; *RA*, resistance arm (perpendicular between axis and RLA); *RLA*, resistance line of action.

3-8). If the weight of the average hand is approximately 0.9 pound, and if lengths of the forearm trough and palmar support are 8 inches and 2½ inches, respectively, the resultant force at the proximal end of the splint may be computed according to the formula

$$F \times FA = RA \times R$$

or

$$F = \frac{R \times RA}{FA}$$
$$= \frac{0.9 \times 2.5}{8}$$
$$= \frac{2.25}{8}$$
$$= 0.28 \text{ pound}$$

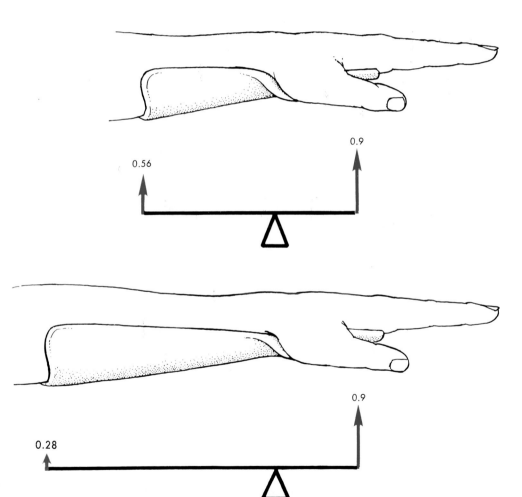

Fig. 3-9. As shown in these scale drawings, the transferred weight of the hand is more comfortably supported by the leverage of a long forearm bar.

If the forearm trough (FA) were only 4 inches in length and the palmar support and resistance remained unchanged, the force at the proximal end of the splint would be twice as great (Fig. 3-9), resulting in patient discomfort and considerably magnifying the chances for pressure problems of the underlying soft tissue:

$$F = \frac{R \times RA}{FA}$$
$$= \frac{0.9 \times 2.5}{4}$$
$$= 0.56 \text{ pound}$$

To simplify the concepts of parallel forces, the splints in Figs. 3-7 to 3-9 are shown in neutral position. Similar concepts apply to any rigid support regardless of shape (Fig. 3-10). If the weight of the hand, its direction of force, and the length of the palmar support are constant, the resulting force at the end of the splint may be decreased by lengthening the forearm trough. This concept may be further generalized to include other types of splints and splint components. Given a constant resistance, resistance line of action, and resistance arm, the amount of force at the opposite end of the first-class lever may be decreased by increasing the length of the force arm (Fig. 3-11).

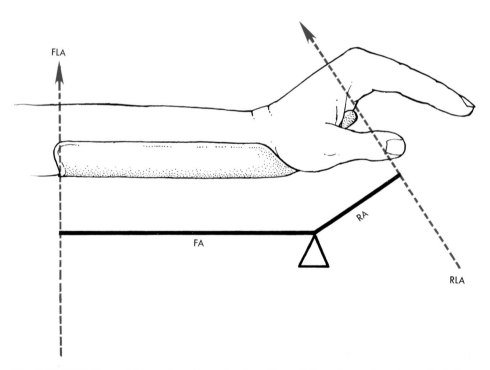

Fig. 3-10. With the wrist bar placed in extension, the splint continues to act as a first-class lever, but the direction of the resistance line of action is altered. *FLA,* Force line of action; *FA,* force arm; *RA,* resistance arm; *RLA,* resistance line of action.

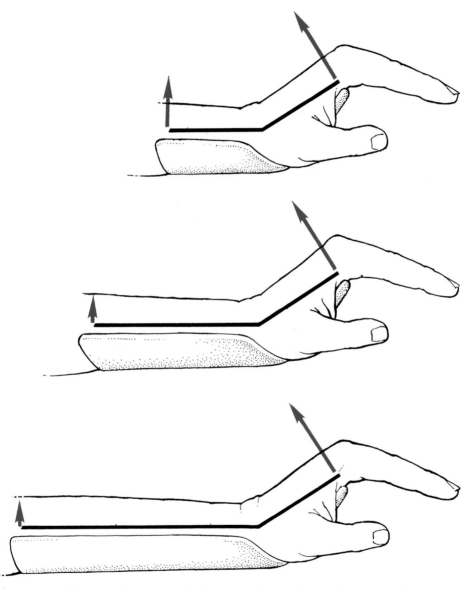

Fig. 3-11. As illustrated in these scale drawings, a longer forearm bar or trough decreases the resultant pressure caused by the proximally transferred weight of the hand to the volar forearm.

The preceding examples indicate the relative relationship between the length of the force arm and the length of the resistance arm, which is designated mechanical advantage (MA):

$$MA = \frac{Force\ arm}{Resistance\ arm}$$

In the previous examples, when the force arm was 8 inches, the mechanical advantage was 3.2, but the mechanical advantage was decreased to 1.6 when the forearm trough was shortened to 4 inches. Splints with greater mechanical advantage will produce less proximal force, resulting in diminished pressure and increased comfort.

Careful control of the force system between splint components will also augment the durability of splints. For example, consider the lever action of an outrigger on the proximal bond or rivet attaching the outrigger to the forearm trough. If the outrigger is viewed as a rigid first-class lever system, the amount of force generated on the proximal attachment may be computed for progressively increased attachment lengths when the resistance, resistance line of action, and resistance arm remain unchanged (Fig. 3-12). A longer force arm will result in

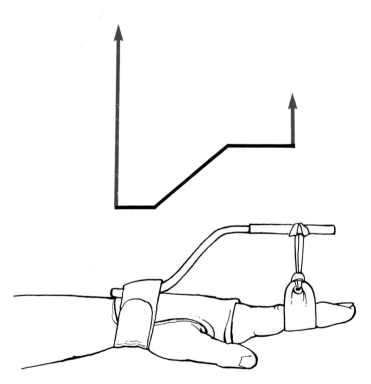

Fig. 3-12. An extended outrigger attachment length produces less leverage on the proximal rivet (drawings to scale).

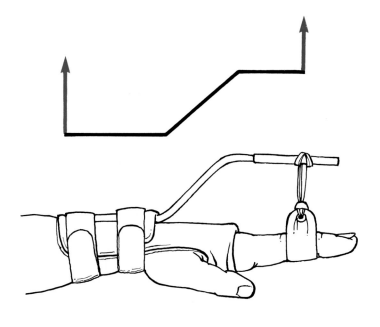

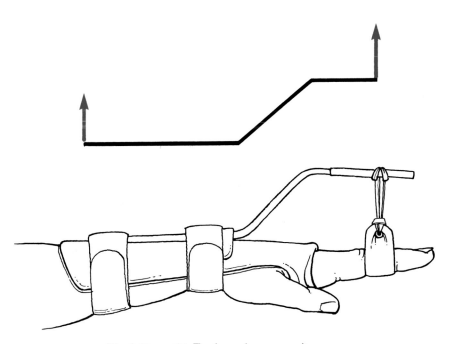

Fig. 3-12, cont'd. For legend see opposite page.

a longer attachment bar and increased mechanical advantage, producing less force on the proximal bond and a stronger, more durable union of the two splint parts.

The combination of the first two mechanical principles supports the common experiential findings that long, wide splints are more comfortable and more durable than are short, narrow ones. When a segment is being splinted, the splint should extend approximately two thirds its length and be contoured to half its width.

Use optimum rotational force. The mobilization of stiffened joints through dynamic traction requires a thorough understanding of the resolution of forces to obtain optimum splint effectiveness without producing patient frustration or increased damage through joint compression or separation.

Theoretically any force applied to a bony segment to mobilize a joint may be resolved into a pair of concurrent rectangular components acting in definite directions. These two components consist of a rotational element producing joint rotation and a translational element producing joint distraction or compression (Fig. 3-13). As a force approximates a perpendicular angle to the segment being mobilized, the translational element is lessened and the rotational component increases until at 90 degrees the full magnitude of the force is applied in a rotational direction (Fig. 3-14). In practical terms this means that dynamic traction should be applied at a 90-degree angle to harness the force potential of the traction device without producing an unwanted pushing or pulling force on the articular surfaces of the involved joint. This also means that, as the passive range of motion of the joint begins to improve, the outrigger to which the traction device

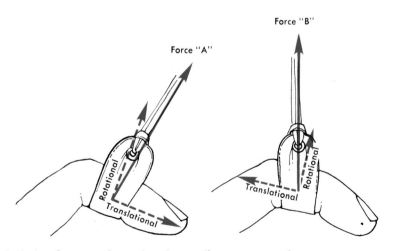

Fig. 3-13. Any force may be analyzed according to rotary and nonrotary components.

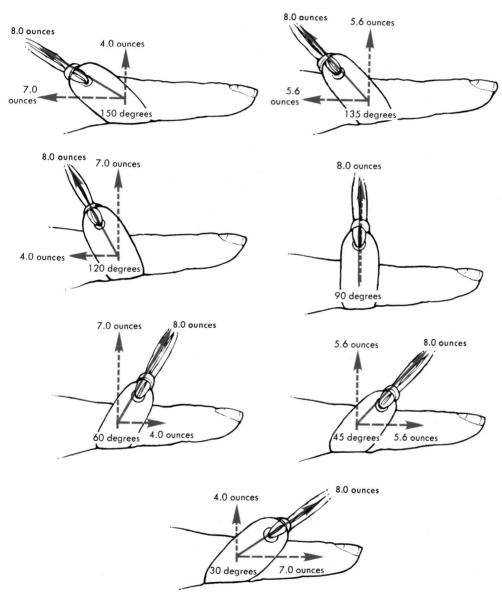

Fig. 3-14. At 90 degrees the translational force is zero, resulting in no element of joint compression or distraction. *Dotted lines,* Rotational force; *dashed lines,* translational force; *solid arrows,* traction assist force.

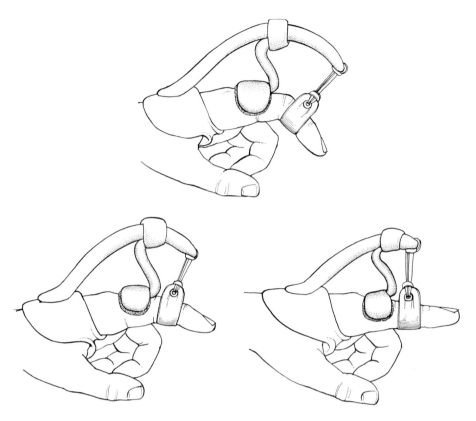

Fig. 3-15. A 90-degree angle of the dynamic assist to the mobilized segment must be maintained as passive joint motion changes.

is attached must be adjusted to maintain the 90-degree angle (Fig. 3-15). In the case of multiple joint splinting, when motion limitations may not be the same, it may be necessary to provide one or more outrigger extensions for adjacent fingers to maintain the required 90-degree angle of pull (Fig. 3-16). Careful attention to the patient's complaints about the splint will provide useful clues as to its mechanical function. If the patient observes that the finger cuffs tend to migrate distally or proximally on the fingers, a 90-degree angle probably has not been achieved or maintained.

An analysis of the interaction between rotational and translational elements may also provide insight as to why some three-point pressure splints such as safety pins and joint jacks become clinically less effective as the flexion angle of the joint is increased (Fig. 3-17). Once again, clinical experience is verified by mechanical force assessment. Because the proximal and distal translational elements produce joint compression with resulting abatement of the rotational components, joint jacks and safety pin splints are more appropriately employed for flexion contractures of 35 degrees or less.

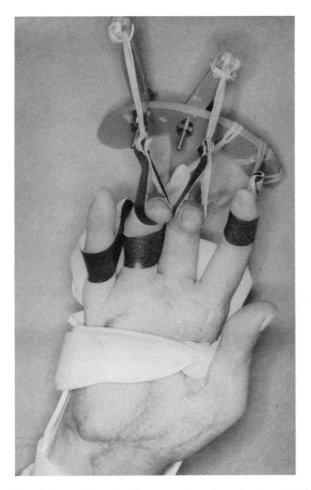

Fig. 3-16. Adaptation of the outrigger is often necessary in order to maintain a perpendicular pull on segments whose passive joint motions are dissimilar.

Consider the torque effect. Torque equals the product of the force times the length of the arm on which it acts ($T = F \times FA$). This concept is important in splinting because the amount of pull from a dynamic assist is not equal to the amount of rotational force or torque at the joint. The amount of torque depends on the distance between the joint axis and the point of attachment of the dynamic assist. The torque increases as the distance between the two increases if the applied force is held constant (Fig. 3-18). This explains why a patient may be able to tolerate a given amount of dynamic traction at one location but cannot tolerate the same amount when the attachment device is moved distally. Patients may be taught to use the torque phenomenon advantageously by advancing their finger cuffs distally as their pain tolerance permits. This must be done judiciously,

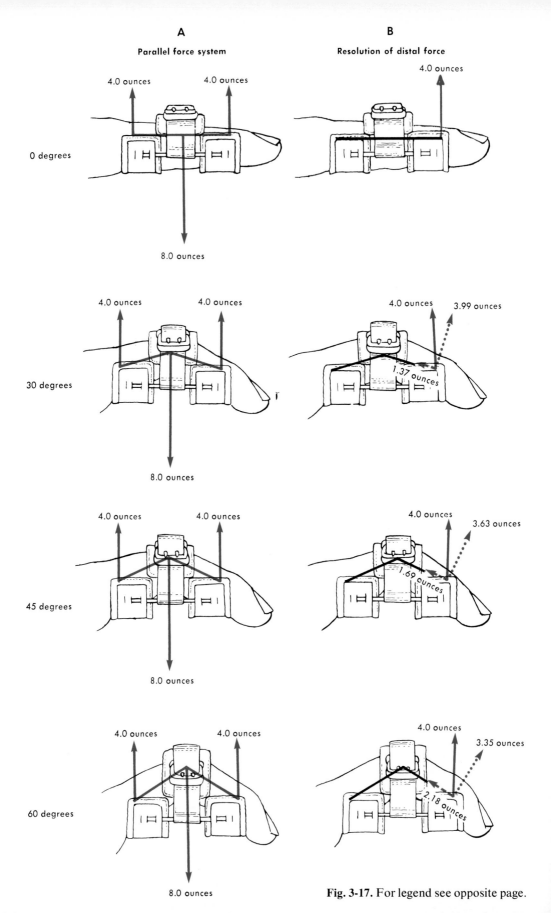

A

Parallel force system

B

Resolution of distal force

0 degrees

4.0 ounces   4.0 ounces

8.0 ounces

4.0 ounces

30 degrees

4.0 ounces   4.0 ounces

8.0 ounces

4.0 ounces   3.99 ounces

1.37 ounces

45 degrees

4.0 ounces   4.0 ounces

8.0 ounces

4.0 ounces   3.63 ounces

1.69 ounces

60 degrees

4.0 ounces   4.0 ounces

8.0 ounces

4.0 ounces   3.35 ounces

2.18 ounces

Fig. 3-17. For legend see opposite page.

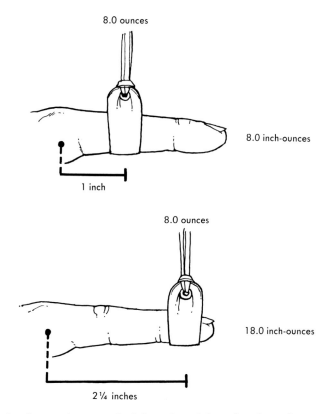

8.0 ounces

8.0 inch-ounces

1 inch

8.0 ounces

18.0 inch-ounces

2 ¼ inches

Fig. 3-18. As the distance between the joint axis and the point of attachment of the dynamic assist increases, the amount of torque on the joint increases.

Fig. 3-17. While the magnitude of the parallel forces of a three-point pressure splint remain constant with the PIP joint in various degrees of flexion (**A**), the rotational and translational components of the proximal and distal forces (only distal end illustrated for simplicity) change until at 60 degrees the compression force (translational) on the joint is nearly two thirds that of the rotational force (**B**). Clinically this means that the greater the flexion deformity the less effective the splint becomes in its ability to correct the deficit. (Key: Dotted arrow = rotational force; dashed arrow = translational force; solid arrow = traction force.) (Special recognition to Kenneth Dunipace, Ph.D., Chairman of the Division of Engineering, Purdue University School of Engineering and Technology at Indianapolis for his assistance with the analysis of this splint.)

however, since too much distal advancement may result in an inferior angle of the traction device or in attenuation of ligamentous structures.

Consider the relative degree of passive mobility of successive joints. When a force is exerted on a proximally based, multiarticular segment, all parts of the segment will be moved in the direction of the force if motion of the successive joints is unimpaired. When motion is limited or stopped at a given articulation, the remaining mobile joints will be moved in the direction of the force with minimal motion occurring at the restricted joint. In other words, when all joints within a longitudinal ray exhibit stiffness, they may be dynamically splinted in unison (Fig. 3-19). If an inequality of passive motion exists, the splint must be adapted to stabilize the normal joints within the segment, allowing the full magnitude of the traction to be directed toward the less mobile joints (Fig. 3-20). If these changes are not made, the rotational force is dissipated in unwanted motion at the mobile joints, resulting in potential damage to the normal joints and ineffective traction on the stiffened joints.

Consider the effects of reciprocal parallel forces. The use of three parallel forces in equilibrium as exemplified by a first-class lever system is basic to splinting of the hand, with the splint acting as the proximal and distal counterforces to the forces of the hand and forearm and a strap at the axis of the splinted segment providing the reciprocal middle force. In an analysis of the interrelationships of forces in a first-class lever system in equilibrium, the combined downward

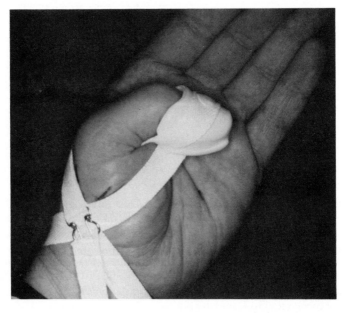

Fig. 3-19. A simple classification splint is appropriate when all joints involved have similar passive range of motion.

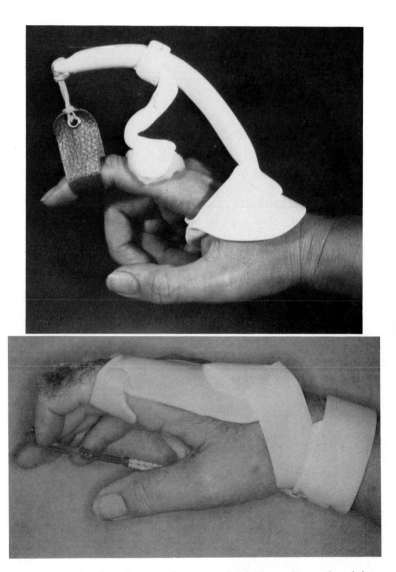

Fig. 3-20. A compound splint allows optimum mechanical purchase when joint motion is unequal within the longitudinal ray.

weights must be opposed by an equal upward force at the axis: A + B = C (Fig. 3-21). This means that the middle opposing force will be of greater magnitude than the force at either the proximal or distal end of the splint. These reciprocal parallel forces form the basis for what is frequently termed *three-point fixation*. Since the middle force in splinting is frequently placed over a joint (Fig. 3-22), care should be taken to minimize the amount of pressure exerted on the underly-

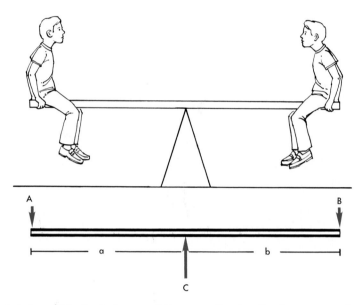

Fig. 3-21. A balanced teeter-totter provides an easily visualized representation of a first-class lever in equilibrium. The combined downward weights (*A* and *B*) must be opposed by an equal opposite force (*C*).

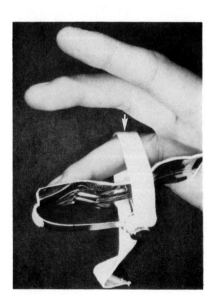

Fig. 3-22. If not monitored carefully, excessive pressure at the site of the middle opposing force (*arrow*) may cause soft tissue damage.

ing soft tissue. This may be accomplished by widening the area of force application.

Understanding parallel force systems also allows the accurate prediction of high-stress areas within the splint itself. Because the summation of the proximal and distal forces equals the middle opposite direction force, it becomes readily apparent why splints with wrist bars frequently become fatigued and fracture at the wrist, and outriggers break at the level of the proximal bend (Fig. 3-23). When

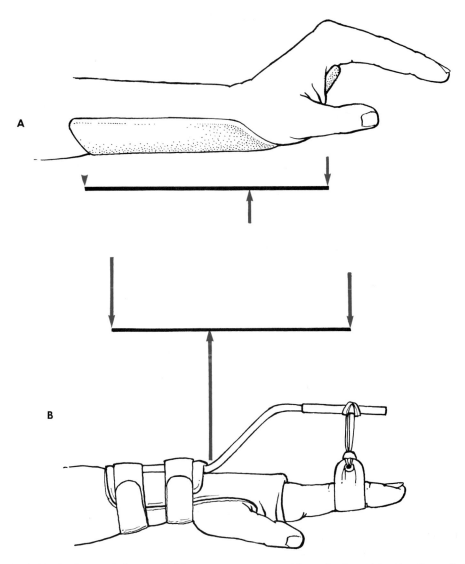

Fig. 3-23. Analyses of the parallel force systems present in a simple wrist extension splint (**A**) and a dorsal outrigger (**B**) indicate the areas of greatest stress to be at the wrist and the proximal bend, respectively.

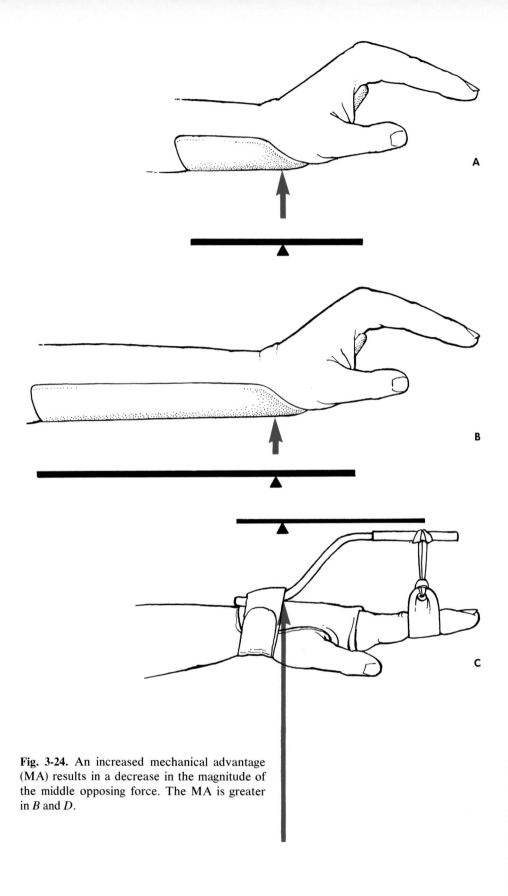

Fig. 3-24. An increased mechanical advantage (MA) results in a decrease in the magnitude of the middle opposing force. The MA is greater in *B* and *D*.

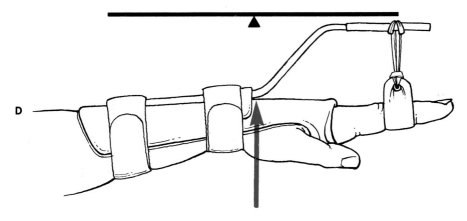

D

Fig. 3-24, cont'd. For legend see opposite page.

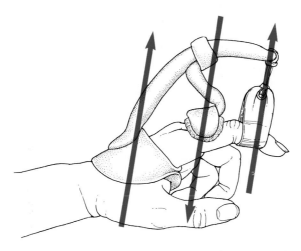

Fig. 3-25. Reciprocal parallel forces may be identified in this compound proximal interphalangeal extension splint.

the mechanical advantage (MA) is increased, the middle opposing force is decreased (Fig. 3-24). Anticipation of the greater magnitude of the middle force allows preventive measures to be taken during the design and construction phases. The forearm bar may be lengthened to decrease the force and the vulnerable area may be contoured or reinforced to increase the mechanical strength of the material.

Another example of reciprocal parallel forces is the force interrelationships within a dorsal outrigger with a lumbrical bar. The lumbrical bar provides a reciprocal middle force to the upward force at the proximal and distal ends of the splint (Fig. 3-25). The resulting downward force at the lumbrical bar is greater than the forces at either end of the splint, further explaining the finding that pres-

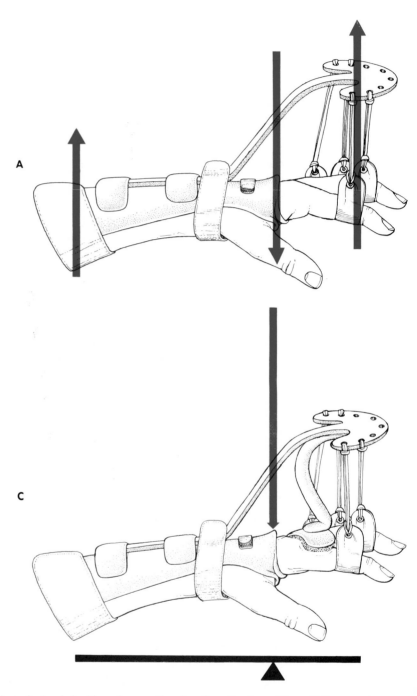

Fig. 3-26. Addition of a lumbrical bar changes the site of application of the middle opposing force (**A** and **B**). Because of an increased mechanical advantage, the force at the lumbrical bar is less than the force at the dorsal metacarpal bar (**C** and **D**).

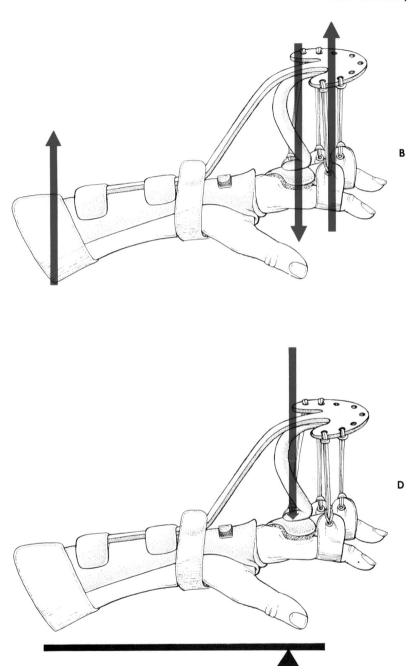

Fig. 3-26, cont'd. For legend see opposite page.

sure is consistently a problem under lumbrical bars and must be dealt with by good fit and dissemination of pressure through padding.

The concept of three-point reciprocal forces may be of further assistance in attempts to eliminate splint pressure over a given area. For example, the middle opposing force on a dorsal outrigger without a lumbrical bar occurs at the distal aspect of the dorsal metacarpal bar, resulting in downward force on the dorsum of the hand. If splint pressure in this area were contraindicated due to edema, poor skin quality, or underlying metacarpal fractures, the addition of a lumbrical bar would change the position of the middle reciprocal force to the dorsum of the proximal phalanx, resulting in rotation upward, away from the dorsum of the hand by the dorsal metacarpal bar (Fig. 3-26, *A* and *B*). The addition of a lumbrical bar also increases the mechanical advantage of the splint and decreases the magnitude of the middle opposing force (Fig. 3-26, *C* and *D*).

Provide contour. The time-honored engineering principle of strength through contour is directly applicable to the design and construction of hand splints and is in many instances a concept that is concomitant with the previous consideration of force dissemination and use of leverage.

When a large force is placed on a flat, thin piece of material, the counterforce produced by the material is insufficient, and the material bends. If, however, the material is contoured into a half-cyclinder shape, the material has, in mechanical terms, become stiffer (Fig. 3-27) and produces a greater counterforce, enabling the material to withstand greater forces without bending (Fig. 3-28).

In considering the design of a splint and the materials to be used, one must take care to match the design to the material properties. The low-temperature materials commonly used in physicians' offices and therapy departments for splint fabrication are easily bendable in sheet form, requiring splint designs that provide strength through contour. The thicker high-temperature plastics and specific

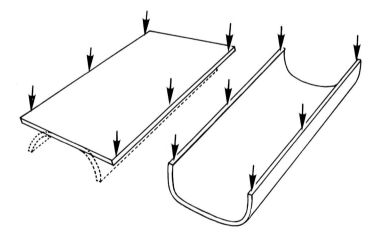

Fig. 3-27. Contour mechanically increases material strength.

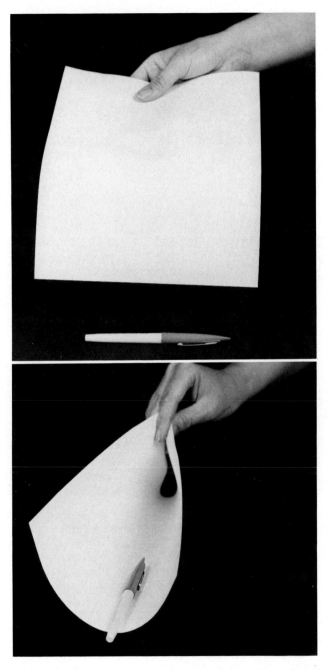

Fig. 3-28. A flat sheet of paper cannot hold the weight of a pen, but, when the paper is contoured into a partial cylinder shape, the pen is supported.

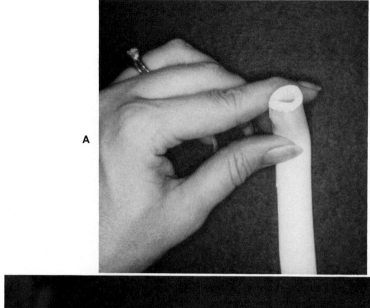

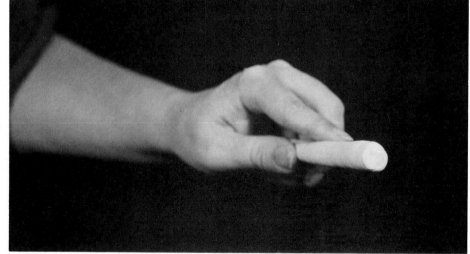

Fig. 3-29. Depending on the specific properties of the low-temperature plastic, outrigger strength may be increased by forming a tube (**A**) or solid coil (**B**).

metals conversely do not need the additional strength attained through material contour and are appropriate for the narrower bar type of splints. Outriggers may be constructed of either kind of material, but, if a low-temperature plastic substance is chosen, mechanical thickness is essential for strength in the form of either a hollow tube or solid coil (Fig. 3-29).

Eliminate friction. Kinetic friction occurs when surfaces in contact with each other move relative to one another. If a difference in density exists between the surfaces, the harder surface may begin to erode the softer, less dense surface, or, if the surfaces are similar, damage may occur on either side or on both sides.

Clinically kinetic friction may occur between the splint and the extremity or between contiguous cutaneous surfaces; in either case it may result in skin irritation, blistering, and eventual breakdown. Friction caused by a splint usually indicates poor fit, improper joint alignment, or inefficient fastening devices. Friction between cutaneous surfaces such as adjacent digits may often be abated by interposing a layer of gauze bandage between the two surfaces. Steps should be taken to alleviate the frictional problem at the first sign of cutaneous embarrassment, since, if the device is left unattended, prolonged trauma to the skin may render the extremity refractory to further splinting efforts until healing occurs.

SUMMARY

Initially the clinician engaged in the preparation of hand splints may consider the mechanical principles of splinting to be technically difficult and not truly germane to the clinical situation. Nonetheless, it is extremely important that the general principles be learned and reviewed so that the finished product is more than an accumulation of the splint maker's experience through numerous inefficient, nonproductive trials. The mathematic details of mechanical engineering or bioengineering are not essential to the basic conceptual understanding of the mechanics of splint design and preparation. A concentrated effort to understand the principles described in this chapter combined with periodic review as experience is gained will pay large dividends in the ultimate performance of a splint.

CHAPTER 4

Fit principles

MECHANICAL CONSIDERATIONS

Use principles of mechanics.
    Reduce pressure
    Use optimum rotational force
    Eliminate friction
    Use optimum leverage

ANATOMIC CONSIDERATIONS

Accommodate bony prominences.
Incorporate dual obliquity concepts.
Consider ligamentous stress.
Maintain arches.
Align splint axis with anatomic axis.
Use skin creases as boundaries.

KINESIOLOGIC CONSIDERATIONS

Allow for kinematic changes.
Employ kinetic concepts.

TECHNICAL CONSIDERATIONS

Develop patient rapport.
Work efficiently.
Change method according to properties of materials used.

The accurate fitting of hand splints to accommodate the individual anatomic variations of patients with a wide variety of clinical problems is a demanding process. Prefabricated splints designed for universal application or poorly contoured splints created without a thorough knowledge of the principles of splint fit will be uncomfortable and result in pressure problems or disuse, often with substantial functional loss to the patient.

With the advent of a wide spectrum of fabrication materials that can be individually adapted to each patient's needs, no excuse can be given for the use of splints that do not fit comfortably and are poorly tolerated. This chapter deals with the principles of splint fitting, which must be thoroughly understood by those engaged in the management of hand problems.

The principles of fitting comprise the second major category in the hierarchy of hand splint conceptualization. These principles encompass mechanical, anatomic, kinesiologic, and technical factors. Fit concepts relating to anatomic structures include consideration of bones, joints, ligaments, arches, and mechanical principles that are directly applied to the shaping of hand splints. Kinesiologic concepts deal with the hand in motion and with the forces that implement this motion, and technical principles incorporate techniques based on practical application and efficiency. The mechanical principles described in Chapter 3 are applied to the fitting of a hand splint, which, when properly done, must incorporate all these concepts to attain ultimate design effectiveness.

MECHANICAL CONSIDERATIONS

Use principles of mechanics. Employment of the principles of mechanics during the fitting of a hand splint is of paramount importance, since the use of improper forces may result in damage to cutaneous, ligamentous, or articular surfaces. In attempting to increase motion of a joint, the force should always be directed perpendicular to both the mobilized segment and the rotational axis of the joint. When traction is applied simultaneously to several joints of the same digital ray, a perpendicular pull must be attained at each rotational axis. Other mechanical principles that must be considered in splint fitting include leverage as applied to the placement of fingernail hooks, dissemination of the applied force to reduce pressure, and elimination of friction. Care should be taken periodically to reevaluate the dynamic forces employed in each splint, and alterations should be incorporated as the pathologic state of the hand changes.

ANATOMIC CONSIDERATIONS
Bone

Accommodate bony prominences. The bony prominences of the extremity must always be considered when fitting a splint. Subcutaneous soft tissue is at a minimum over these areas, rendering them more vulnerable to externally applied pressure. Improper contouring of the splint material may cause pressure ischemia, which often results in tissue necrosis.

In the upper extremity the most common problematic bony prominences include the ulnar styloid process, the pisiform, the radial styloid process, the heads of the metacarpals, and the base of the first metacarpal (Fig. 4-1). Caution must be employed when fitting parts of splints that come into contact with or are adjacent to these bony prominences, such as forearm bars or troughs, opponens bars, wrist bars, lumbrical bars, and dorsal metacarpal bars. Care should be taken to either avoid these protuberances or to decrease the pressure over them by widening the area of application through increased material contact or the use of selective padding (Fig. 4-2).

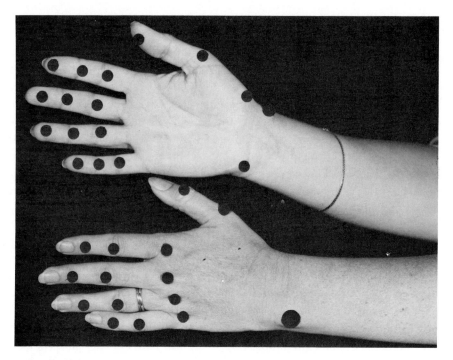

Fig. 4-1. Pressure over bony prominences may cause soft tissue damage.

Incorporate dual obliquity concepts. Dual obliquity is a second important consideration in splint fitting that is determined by the skeletal configuration of the hand. This principle has two anatomic ramifications: the progressive decrease of length of the metacarpals from the radial to the ulnar aspect of the hand and the immobility of the second and third metacarpals as compared to the mobile first, fourth, and fifth metacarpals. Due to this unique structural formation, two oblique lines may be drawn that particularly relate to splint design and fit. The first, from a dorsal aspect, shows the progressive metacarpal shortening (Fig. 4-3); the second, from a distal transverse view, clarifies the progressive metacarpal descent from the radial to the ulnar side of the normal hand in a resting posture (Fig. 4-4).

Functionally, this anatomic arrangement means that, with the forearm fully supinated and resting on a table, a straight object gripped comfortably in the hand will not be parallel to the table but will be slightly higher on the radial side. When the wrist is held in a nondeviated posture, the object will also not be held perpendicular to the longitudinal axis of the forearm but will form an oblique angle from the proximal ulnar aspect of the hand to the radial aspect distally.

This principle of dual obliquity must then be translated to any splint part that supports or incorporates the second through fifth metacarpal bones. That is, a

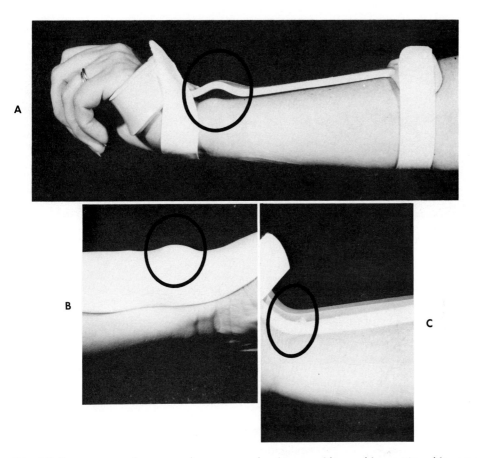

Fig. 4-2. Pressure over bony prominences may be decreased by avoidance (**A**), wider area of contact (**B**), or padding (**C**).

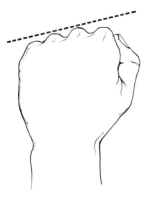

Fig. 4-3. Dorsally, the consecutive metacarpal heads create an oblique angle to the longitudinal axis of the forearm.

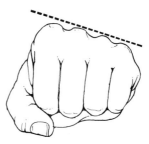

Fig. 4-4. Distally, the fisted hand exhibits an ulnar metacarpal descent that creates an oblique angle in the transverse plane of the forearm.

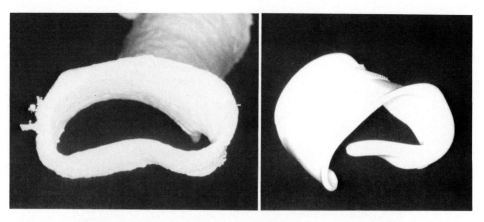

Fig. 4-5. The metacarpal bars should be slightly higher on the radial side when viewed distally.

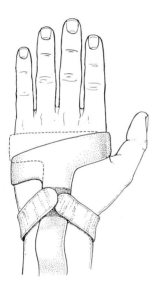

Fig. 4-6. The metacarpal bars should follow the oblique configuration of the metacarpal heads. *Solid lines,* Correct; *broken line,* incorrect.

splint must be longer and higher on the radial side (Fig. 4-5) and at no time should end or bend perpendicular to the longitudinal axis of the forearm when the wrist is not deviated to either side (Fig. 4-6).

Ligaments

Consider ligamentous stress. The preservation of ligamentous structures in correct position and tension is another anatomic principle used in effective fitting

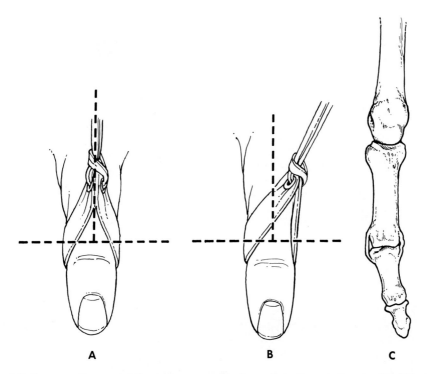

Fig. 4-7. Correct alignment (**A**). A nonperpendicular pull to the rotational axis of the joint (**B**) will produce unequal stress on the collateral ligaments (**C**).

of hand splints. Since ligaments normally provide for joint stability and direction, it is important that their functions be considered when attempting to augment hand function with splinting devices.

From a simplistic point of view, each metacarpophalangeal and interphalangeal joint has three similar ligaments whose presence directly influences the construction of hand splints: two collateral ligaments and a volar plate ligament. In hinged joints, such as the interphalangeal joints, the collateral ligaments prevent joint mobility in the coronal plane, that is, ulnar and radial deviation. Because of this anatomic arrangement, it is important that splints designed to dynamically mobilize these joints be constructed so that their line of pull is perpendicular to the joint axis (Fig. 4-7). Static splints must also be designed to protect this ligamentous support system so that instability does not result. It is believed that after digital injury, which requires proximal interphalangeal joint immobilization, a splint that maintains the joint in near-full extension will best preserve collateral ligament length and prevent flexion contracture. It is also important to monitor splints carefully as passive joint motion improves so that ligamentous structures are not overstretched.

Because of the camlike structure of the heads of the metacarpals, the collateral

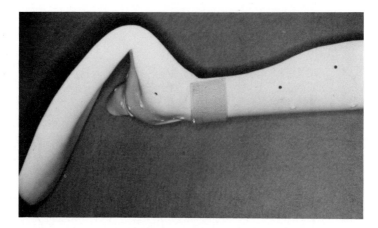

Fig. 4-8. This safe position splint maintains the metacarpophalangeal joints in flexion and the interphalangeal joints in extension.

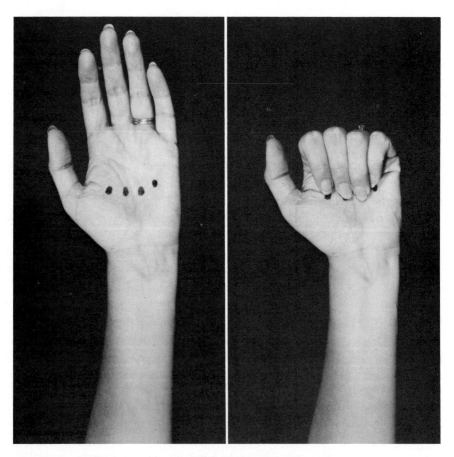

Fig. 4-9. Digital palmar contact occurs from the middle of the first metacarpal to the hypothenar eminence when the fingers are flexed simultaneously.

ligaments of the metacarpophalangeal joints are not taut until the proximal phalanx is brought into full flexion, allowing finger abduction-adduction in extension and limited lateral motion when the fingers are flexed. This is an important concept to recognize when fitting splints that act on the metacarpophalangeal joints. If the full length of the collateral ligaments of the metacarpophalangeal joints is not maintained, a loss of flexion may occur, and the ensuing fixed contracture may be impossible to improve by conservative means. So-called safe position splints, such as the Michigan burn splint (Fig. 4-8), embody this concept by positioning the metacarpophalangeal joints in flexion to maintain collateral ligament length. More difficult to envision, but equally important, is the action of a lumbrical bar that determines the degree of extension allowed the metacarpophalangeal joints. If the potential for metacarpophalangeal joint stiffness is present, the lumbrical bar should be adjusted to hold the proximal phalanges in near-full flexion.

When the fingers are individually flexed, the tips of the digits will touch the palm in a small area near the thenar crease. However, when the fingers are flexed simultaneously, digital palmar contact will occur from the middle of the first metacarpal to the hypothenar eminence (Fig. 4-9). Functionally this allows the hand to grasp objects without the fingers overlapping each other. The length of the metacarpophalangeal joint collateral ligaments is critical to this digital spreading; in splinting this length must be preserved when dynamically augmenting passive

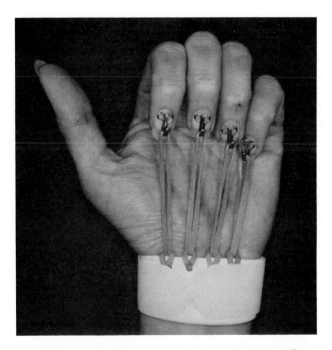

Fig. 4-10. To maintain the necessary metacarpophalangeal collateral ligament length to allow simultaneous finger flexion, dynamic flexion assists should not overlap at the level of the wrist.

flexion. At the wrist level, the proximal ends of the traction devices should not be anchored at a single point, but should individually originate, thereby permitting digital separation (Fig. 4-10).

Volar plate ligaments function to prevent hyperextension of the metacarpophalangeal and interphalangeal joints of the hand. When employing dynamic devices to increase passive joint extension, such as outriggers, serial cylinder casts, or safety pin splints, caution should be taken to prevent attenuation of these structures. This may be done by tension adjustment and by careful monitoring of the progress of the joint as it is brought to the neutral position (Fig. 4-11).

The thumb carpometacarpal joint is a saddle articulation that allows motion of the first metacarpal through all planes. There are five primary thumb carpometacarpal ligaments; when fitting thumb splints, one should give careful thought to the position in which the thumb is placed and the ultimate functional ramifications of this position. Maintenance of the first web space must be emphasized, and for most supportive or positioning splints the thumb should be held in wide abduction.

Arches

Maintain arches. The three skeletal arches of the hand (proximal transverse, distal transverse, and longitudinal) must also be taken into consideration in attaining congruous splint fit. The distal transverse or metacarpal arch consists of an immobile center post, the second and third metacarpal heads, around which the mobile first, fourth, and fifth metacarpals rotate (Fig. 4-12). The longitudinal arch (Fig. 4-13) on a sagittal plane embodies the carpals, metacarpals, and pha-

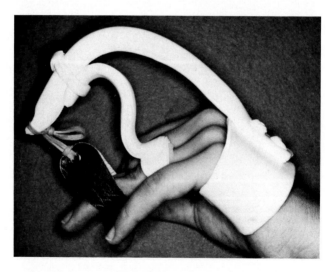

Fig. 4-11. Attenuation of the volar plate with resultant hyperextension of the joint may occur with prolonged unsupervised extension traction.

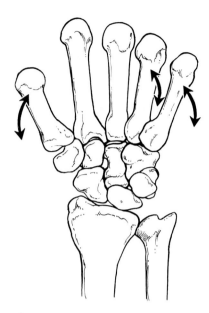

Fig. 4-12. The mobile first, fourth, and fifth metacarpals allow the hand to assume an anteriorly concave configuration, which is fundamental to coordinated grasp.

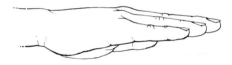

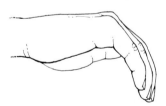

Fig. 4-13. In the sagittal plane the motion potential of the segments comprising the longitudinal arch is approximately 280 degrees.

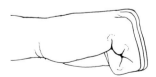

langes and allows approximately 280 degrees of total active motion in each finger. The carpal or proximal transverse arch, although existent anatomically, is of secondary importance in splinting because the flexor tendons and volar neurovascular structures that traverse through the arch obliterate its concavity exteriorly. These arches, which combine stability and flexibility, allow the normal hand to grasp an almost endless array of items of various sizes and shapes with a maximum or minimum of surface contact.

To maintain the maximum potential mobility of the hand, the distal transverse and longitudinal arches must be preserved throughout the duration of treatment. The distal transverse arch should be apparent in any splint that incorporates the metacarpals (Fig. 4-14), provided significant dorsal and volar swelling is not present. If this type of edema exists, care should be taken to adjust the parts of the splint that are responsible for supporting the arch as the edema subsides. Care should also be taken to continue the transverse arch configuration in splint parts that extend distal to the metacarpophalangeal joints such as lumbrical bars or finger pans (Fig. 4-15).

Because of the mobility afforded by the longitudinal arch, splints that affect it are varied. Basically, any splint that incorporates the phalanges, either statically or dynamically, influences the state of this arch. The use of a finger pan, either in a

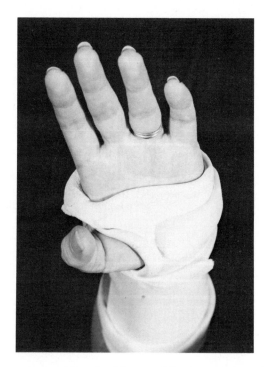

Fig. 4-14. The metacarpal bar should support the transverse metacarpal arch.

resting pan splint or a safe position splint, statically provides support for the entire length of the longitudinal arch. Extension or flexion outriggers, metacarpopha- langeal flexion cuffs, and elastic traction applied through the use of fingernail clips are examples of splint parts that dynamically augment the passive range of motion of the longitudinal arch. When fitting splints that support only certain segments of the longitudinal arch, care must be taken not to block the motion of the remaining components of the arch, either distally or proximally. This may be done through careful attention to the dorsal and volar skin creases and their relationships to each end of the splint (Fig. 4-16). Whenever support of any part of the longitudinal arch is to be achieved, the desired position of the involved metacarpophalangeal and interphalangeal joints must be predetermined before fitting may commence. This determination is dependent on the specific purpose of application of the splint and the individual hand condition with which one is dealing.

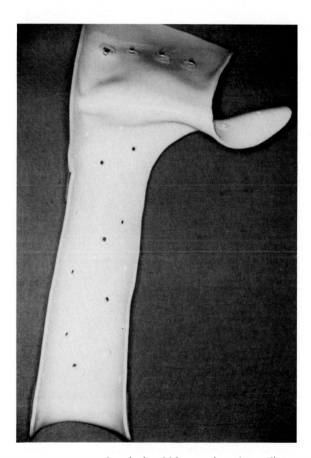

Fig. 4-15. The transverse metacarpal arch should be continued to splint parts that affect the fingers.

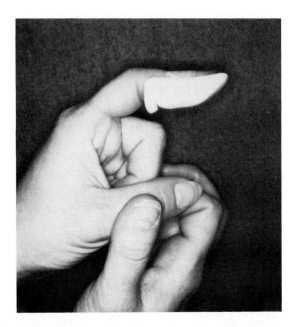

Fig. 4-16. Care should be taken not to impede motion of unsplinted segments of the longitudinal arch.

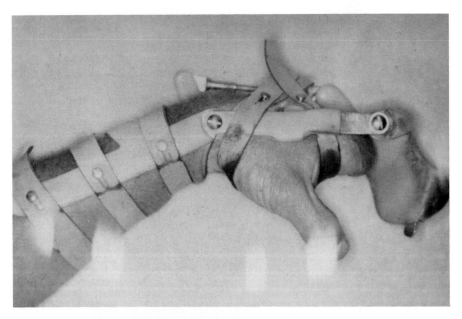

Fig. 4-17. The rotational axis of the splint must be correctly aligned with the anatomic rotational axis of the joint to allow unhampered simultaneous movement of both joints. This partial hand prosthesis exhibits good alignment at the wrist joint. (Splint by Lawrence Czap, O.T.R., orthotist, Columbus, Ohio.)

Joints

Two principles prevail when fitting splints that are designed to mobilize joints through dynamic traction: achievement of the correct alignment of the splint axis with the anatomic joint axis and use of a 90-degree angle that is also perpendicular to the rotational axis of the joint.

Align splint axis with anatomic axis. Articulated splints (Fig. 4-17) must provide correct splint and joint alignment to allow achievement of full motion of the joint being splinted. If this is not accomplished, the splint may not only prove ineffective in increasing motion, but may actually limit joint range. The approximate location of a specific anatomic joint axis may be found through observation of the joint as it moves in the plane in which it is to be splinted.

Use optimum rotational force. When employing dynamic traction to increase the passive range of motion of a joint, the splint should be fitted to eliminate all translational forces and permit only rotational force in the desired plane. This is accomplished by positioning the distal end of the dorsal or volar outrigger at a point that would allow the dynamic assist, such as a rubber band, to pull at a 90-degree angle on the bone to be mobilized. This pull should also be perpendicular to the rotational axis of the joint so that the supporting ligamentous structures are equally stressed. If a 90-degree angle of pull is not employed, and if the force is applied in the direction of the joint, significant pressure may be imparted to the cartilaginous surfaces of the joint as a result of compression of the two bones. If the force is directed away from the joint to be mobilized, the joint surfaces may be distracted, and the patient will have difficulty keeping the traction cuffs on the fingers. As the joint range of motion improves, the length of the outrigger must be changed to accommodate a continuous 90-degree angle of pull (Fig. 4-18).

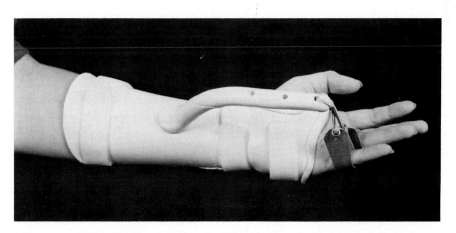

Fig. 4-18. As the finger position changes, the length of the outrigger must be altered to accommodate a 90-degree angle of the traction assist to the segment being mobilized. This volar outrigger is designed to allow the patient to adjust the traction assist.

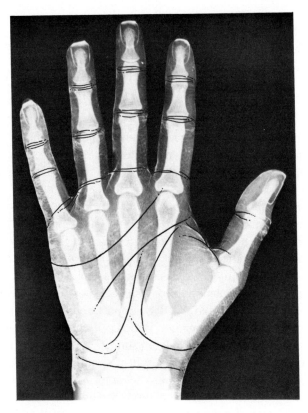

Fig. 4-19. Skin creases correspond directly to underlying joints indicating the boundaries of motion for each segment. (NOTE: Although this is a palmar view, the dye outlines the fingernails and shows through from the dorsum.)

Skin

Concepts of fitting splints with regard to the cutaneous surfaces of the hand include the consideration of skin creases and mechanical principles regarding the dissemination of pressure, elimination of friction, and use of optimum leverage.

Use skin creases as boundaries. Since the dorsal and volar skin creases correspond directly to the underlying joints (Fig. 4-19), their presence graphically indicates the areas at which motion takes place in the hand and provides tangible boundaries for splint preparation. If the metacarpophalangeal joints are to be unencumbered by a splint, the distal aspect of the splint must not be applied beyond the distal palmar flexion crease; if the thumb is to retain full mobility, the splint material should not lie radial to the thenar crease; and full mobility of a proximal interphalangeal joint may be achieved by terminating the splint slightly proximal to the middle flexion crease of the digit. Conversely, if a joint is to be immobilized, the splint should be extended as close as possible to the next seg-

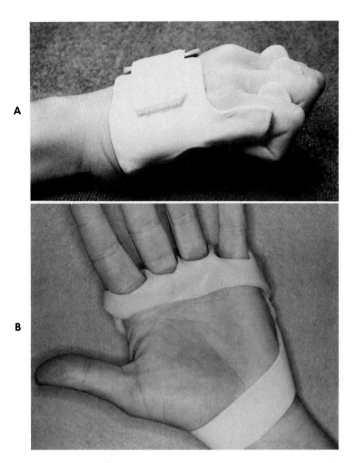

Fig. 4-20. Immobilization or blocking components should be extended to include at least two-thirds the length of the proximal and distal segments that the splint incorporates. **A,** Flexion of the metacarpophalangeal joints is blocked because the volar phalangeal bar is of sufficient length. **B,** This phalangeal bar was not fitted far enough distally and thus allows metacarpophalangeal flexion. (**A** courtesy K. P. MacBain, O.T.R., Vancouver, British Columbia.)

mental crease, both proximally and distally, to provide maximum mechanical purchase (Fig. 4-20).

Use principles of mechanics

Reduce pressure. The dissemination of pressure is another important concept in the design and fitting of hand splints. Excessive pressure, regardless of good splint design and construction, may render the splint intolerable and unwearable. Pressure may be decreased by increasing the area of application. This should be considered in the original design of the splint and may be augmented at the time of

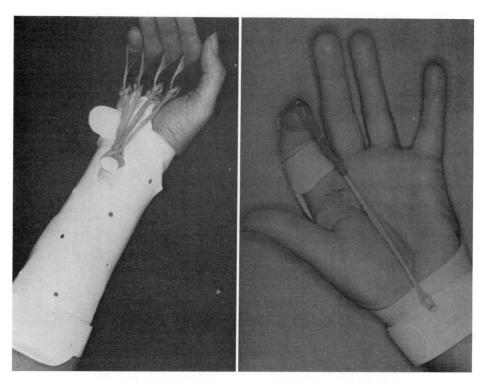

Fig. 4-21. Edge pressure may be decreased by rolling the proximal and distal ends of the splint.

fitting by rolling the proximal and distal ends of the splint (Fig. 4-21) and contouring the material nearly to the full length of the segment being fitted. Padding may also be used appropriately to decrease the influence of splint parts that cannot be widened because of their specific functions or place of application. However, one should beware of the overuse of padding because, in addition to its eventual contamination by moisture and dirt, it is frequently indicative of a poorly fitted splint.

Cutting holes in splints to alleviate pressure is a common mistake that can result in greater pressure around the circumferential border of the cutout with potential tissue injury. It is important to follow the contours of the extremity as closely as possible; if full wound coverage is not present, the splint may be applied over an appropriate dressing. In some instances, application of a splint would be detrimental to specific local tissue viability. The splint should then be designed to avoid this area and any adjacent tissue that might be of questionable viability. The splint border encroaching on this defect should be contoured outward to increase the area of application and decrease the edge pressure (Fig. 4-22).

Eliminate friction. The elimination of friction is the third principle associated

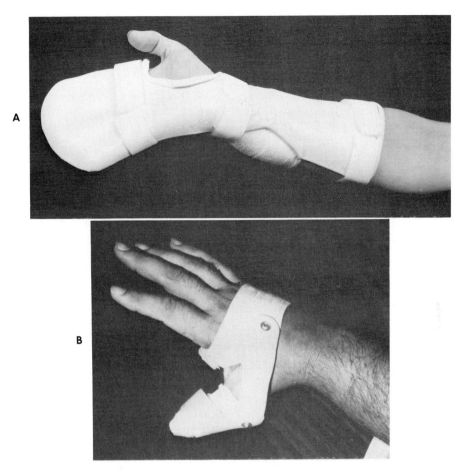

Fig. 4-22. Splint edges that must be adjacent to areas of soft tissue of questionable viability should be contoured outward to decrease pressure. (**B** courtesy Joan Farrell, O.T.R., Lauderhill, Florida.)

with skin. Friction of the splint material against the skin or friction caused by skin against skin, as with adjacent fingers, often is the result of an improperly designed or poorly fitted splint. The splint may be too large, the angle of pull incorrect, or the splint axis may not correspond to the anatomic joint axis. A careful observation of the area of friction and a reevaluation of the various principles of fitting hand splints will probably uncover the problem. Placement of an appropriate material between two cutaneous surfaces may also alleviate troublesome contact areas (Fig. 4-23). Initially, patients should be instructed to remove their splints every 2 to 3 hours to check for areas of skin embarrassment.

Optimum leverage. Fingernail attachment devices such as dress hooks or Velcro buttons should be applied to the proximal and center aspect of the nail. Distal

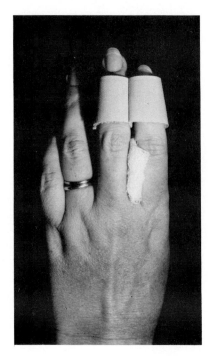

Fig. 4-23. Placement of gauze between two adjacent cutaneous surfaces will decrease friction.

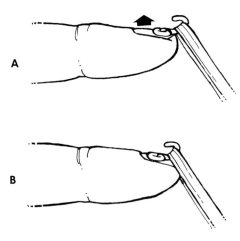

Fig. 4-24. Care should be taken to minimize the leverage effect of a fingernail attachment device on a fingernail bed by avoiding distal attachment. **A,** Incorrect. **B,** Correct.

attachment results in considerable discomfort because of the leverage effect of the nail away from the proximal nail bed (Fig. 4-24).

KINESIOLOGIC CONSIDERATIONS

Kinesiologic considerations encompass two additional concepts pertaining to the actual shaping of a hand splint: kinematic principles and kinetic principles. Kinematic principles deal with the differences between the hand at rest and the hand in motion, and kinetic principles concern the dynamic force relationship between the hand and the splint. Both the design and form of a hand splint should reflect an understanding of these two major concepts.

Allow for kinematic changes. As the fingers and thumb move through an arc of motion from a fully extended position to an attitude of full flexion, basic external anatomic configurations change their relationships. In flexion, volar skin creases approximate, arches deepen, dorsal bony prominences become more apparent, the dorsal surface area elongates, and the palmar length lessens. As the thenar and hypothenar masses move volarly in opposition, the breadth of the hand changes to become convex dorsally and concave volarly, resulting in the increase of dorsometacarpal surface area. A splint designed to allow motion must be fitted to accommodate anticipated changes in the arches and bony prominences. For example, finger extension cuffs must be cut to permit full proximal and distal phalangeal flexion (Fig. 4-25), whereas the entire width of flexion cuffs may be preserved to decrease pressure. Hypothenar bars should not inhibit motion of the

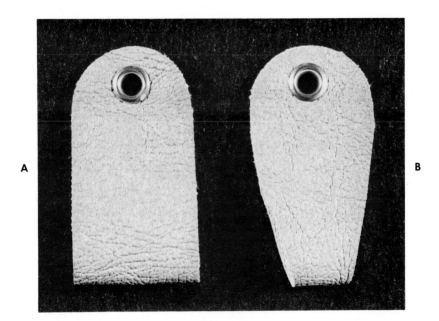

Fig. 4-25. Depending on hand size, extension finger cuffs (**B**) should be cut to allow finger flexion. Flexion cuffs may be used without alteration (**A**).

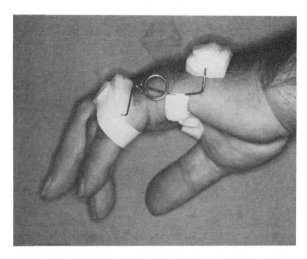

Fig. 4-26. This lumbrical bar prevents metacarpophalangeal joint hyperextension and allows the excursion of extrinsic extensors to be focused on the interphalangeal joints.

first metacarpal, and phalangeal bars should allow unencumbered motion of the segments they do not support. If these types of adaptations are not executed, motion of the hand may be inhibited, pressure and friction injury of the skin may occur, and the splint may be rendered ineffective.

Employ kinetic concepts. The actual positioning of specific splint parts will augment or retard muscle action. An extension finger cuff placed on the proximal phalanx assists the long extensor tendons; interossei and lumbrical forces are reinforced when the cuff is positioned at the middle phalanx. The fitting of a lumbrical bar to prevent metacarpal hyperextension augments extension of the fingers by maximizing the extrinsic extensor action at the interphalangeal joints (Fig. 4-26). Because of the relative lengths of the extrinsic digital flexors and extensors, a wrist bar fitted for extension enhances finger flexion, and conversely a flexed wrist bar favors finger extension. A knowledge of kinetic principles as they pertain to the hand is important in achieving the full potential of splints to increase hand function.

TECHNICAL CONSIDERATIONS

Numerous techniques of fitting hand splints exist that are based on practical everyday experiences. These additional clinical considerations will help increase efficiency and make the fitting process run more smoothly.

Develop patient rapport. An explanation about the proposed splint—its functions, material, and method of forming—implement the development of patient rapport and trust. A rehearsal of the desired position in which the hand is to be splinted before the actual application of the splint material also expedites the fitting process. If thermal materials are used, the patient should be warned that the material will feel warm. Allowing a child to play with scraps of the material before fitting commences is ultimately well worth the extra time and effort!

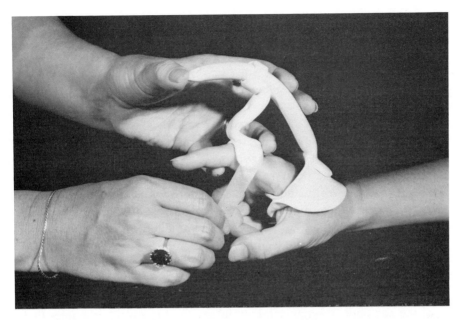

Fig. 4-27. Tape may be used to maintain splint position until plastic hardens.

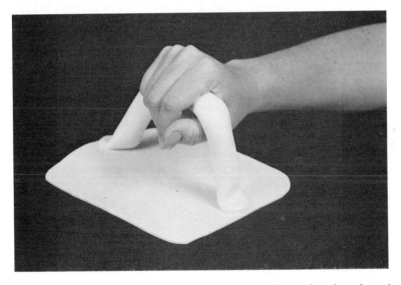

Fig. 4-28. A positioning device may be of assistance when the curing phase is prolonged.

Work efficiently. The use of devices or methods that increase the efficiency of the molding time may also be of considerable benefit. Lightly wrapping a warmed, low-temperature, thermal material splint to the patient's hand and forearm with an Ace bandage allows for full attention to be directed to the positioning of the hand. Strategically applied tape will hold splint parts in position as they cool (Fig. 4-27), and, in working with more slowly setting materials such as plaster, the employment of a hand rest or positioning device (Fig. 4-28) lessens muscle fatigue during the cooling phase.

Allowing gravitational forces to augment splint fabrication is another efficiency consideration of fit. If the splint is to be worn volarly, molding is facilitated by placing the forearm and hand in supination; a dorsal splint will be best fitted in pronation.

Change method according to properties of materials used. Different materials require the use of diverse approaches to the forming procedure. For example, if a protective Stockinette is used during the shaping of a splint constructed of high-temperature material, the resulting splint will be somewhat large for the unprotected hand, requiring further adjustment. Moisture should be eliminated from the surfaces of a material requiring wet heat before application to the patient, and the use of a separating substance such as petroleum jelly augments the removal of newly applied cylindrical plaster splints.

SUMMARY

Those involved in the splinting process must arm themselves with a knowledge of the anatomic, mechanical, kinesiologic, and technical principles that are an absolute prerequisite for proper fit. Failure to adhere to these principles will often result in embarrassing pressure areas, splint disuse, and patient distrust, with the probable attendant decrease of hand function.

The decision to use a splint on the hand of a particular patient is a serious consideration involving the physician and the therapist; a close communication between the two must exist so that the exact function expected from each splint can be realized. If the proper fit techniques are employed, the opportunity for maximum hand function and patient satisfaction is provided.

CHAPTER 5

Construction principles

Strive for good cosmetic effect.
Use equipment appropriate to material.
Use type of heat and temperature appropriate to material.
Use safety precautions.
Round corners.
Smooth edges.
Analyze mechanical principles.
Stabilize joined surfaces.
Finish rivets.
Provide ventilation as necessary.
Secure padding.
Secure straps.

Once a splint has been designed and a pattern prepared, construction is often of less difficulty than the preceding stages and those to follow. The principles of construction represent concepts that are directly applicable to the durability, cosmesis, and comfort of the finished product. Adherence to the twelve principles listed at the beginning of this chapter should produce a splint that will be well tolerated, durable, and visually acceptable.

The construction of a splint may be divided into five phases: (1) transfer of the pattern to the material, (2) heating of the material, (3) cutting of the material, (4) joining of separate parts, and (5) finishing details of the splint. Because fitting of the splint usually occurs after the cutting, there is an obligatory time separation between the initial construction phases and the joining and finishing phases. Many of the principles of construction are applicable to more than one phase and should be considered as overall guidelines rather than as techniques specific to a single phase.

Strive for good cosmetic effect. Since a splint is an extraneous piece of equipment, it has little cosmetic value however well designed, constructed, or fitted it may be. It is therefore important that all efforts be directed toward making the external appearance of the splint as pleasing as is possible. Splints that resemble an aberrant assortment of discarded junk have no place in the present-day thera-

119

peutic armamentarium. Material or fabrication expense should not significantly influence splint cosmesis. Inexpensive materials can often be neatly assembled into a functional splint, and more costly materials may be poorly assembled with resultant splint discoloration, fatigue, and irregular surfaces. Good splint appearance may be achieved through careful attention to detail during the various phases of construction.

Materials should not be overworked. Bubbles and burn spots from overheating are unacceptable, as is the presence of rough edges, sharp corners, pen marks, fingerprints, and dirty smudges. The number of different materials used in a splint should be kept to a minimum, and, when joining pieces of a similar material whose opposing surfaces differ in texture, care should be taken to align the surfaces so that the external surface textures match (Fig. 5-1).

Use equipment appropriate to material. The use of a variety of materials enhances the potential for effective conservative treatment of pathologic hand conditions through splinting techniques, but the use of dissimilar materials creates the necessity of adapting construction methods and equipment to the particular material requirements. This is especially important when switching between low and high temperature–forming substances. For example, a water-insoluble marking device should be used when transferring a pattern to a material that requires wet

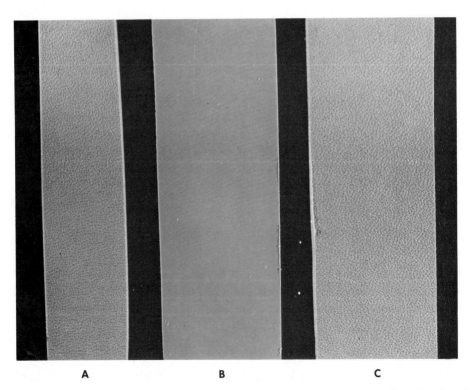

| A | B | C |

Fig. 5-1. Matching textured surfaces improves splint cosmesis. *Correct combination,* **A** and **C**; *incorrect,* **A** and **B** or **B** and **C**.

heat for cutting and forming, whereas the use of a water-soluble pen with a dry heat material is advantageous because the pen marks may be washed off when no longer needed. Although metal files or an electric sander can be used for edge smoothing of high temperature–material splints, these devices cause friction gumming and exaggerate roughness on low temperature–material edges. Power saws produce burrs on the edges of cold, low temperature–forming materials, whereas cutting the same material with scissors after it is warmed produces a continuous, smooth-finished splint edge.

Use type of heat and temperature appropriate to materal. The reaction of splinting materials to heat varies with the type of material, but temperature extremes in either direction (too much heat or not enough) may influence construction techniques. Overheating causes blistering, stretching, and surface irregularities; underheating may produce rough-cut edges and an inequality of pliability. Bonding of low-temperature materials is also not as reliable when the temperature is not at optimum level.

Splint construction may be influenced by the type of heat used. Some materials, such as Orthoplast, bond more readily to themselves when dry heat is employed, eliminating both the possible surface contamination caused by wet heat and the need for additional cleaning with chemical solvents (Fig. 5-2). The type of

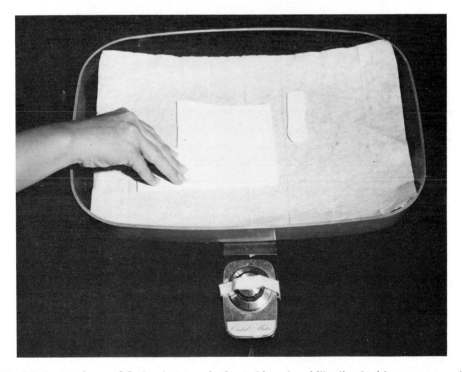

Fig. 5-2. Large pieces of Orthoplast may be heated in a dry skillet lined with a paper towel to prevent sticking and surface impregnation. Use of a dry skillet allows the material temperature to be consistently maintained over several hours, providing malleable plastic whenever it is needed.

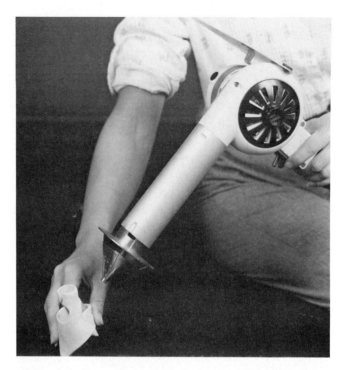

Fig. 5-3. A heat gun and a spot heater direct dry heat to small areas.

heat may also influence the speed at which the material becomes malleable. Most low-temperature materials will respond more quickly and uniformly to wet heat. However, if only a small section of a splint needs heating (Fig. 5-3), the use of dry heat from a heat gun will allow adjacent structures to remain unaltered.

Use safety precautions. Exposure to a large volume of hand trauma patients results in an awareness of the potential dangers of working with both manual and power tools and an appreciation of the need for high safety standards. Eyes should be protected, rings removed, and loose hair and clothing secured (Fig. 5-4) before any piece of power equipment is turned on. Because studies have shown that dull or poorly maintained tools cause accidents, both hand and power tools should be inspected and repaired routinely, with careful attention directed to the wiring of wet-heat electrical appliances.

Protection of the patient and the therapist from potential harm by sharp or hot materials during splint formation and construction stages is also of considerable importance. Gloves and stockinettes provide a heat barrier when working with high-temperature substances, and sharp edges of metal and wire should be taped to prevent inadvertent injury. Materials warmed with wet heat should be dried thoroughly before handling and application.

Round corners. Both inside and outside corners of a splint should be rounded

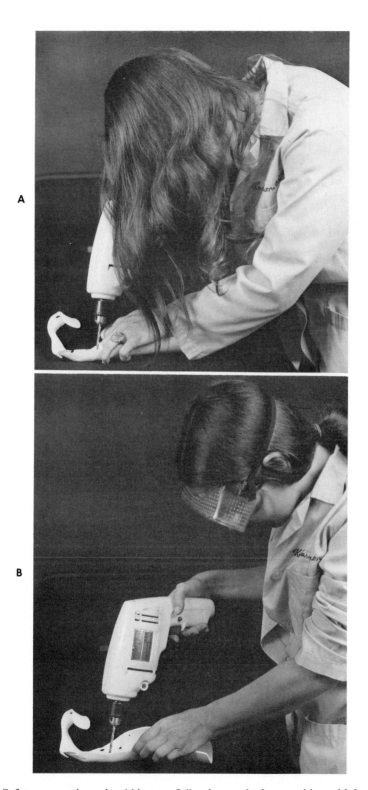

Fig. 5-4. Safety precautions should be carefully observed when working with hand tools or power equipment. **A,** Incorrect. **B,** Correct.

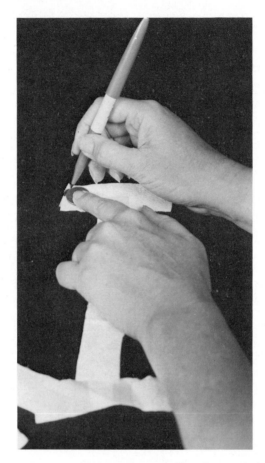

Fig. 5-5. Splint cosmesis is improved if corners are uniformly rounded. This may be accomplished during the transfer stage by drawing around a coin on both external and internal corners.

for increased strength, durability, cosmesis, and comfort. Uniformity of the curves may be attained by drawing around a coin at each corner during the transfer phase of splint construction (Fig. 5-5). Corners should also be rounded on straps and accessory splint parts such as outriggers and finger cuffs (Fig. 5-6).

   Smooth edges. Splint edges should be smoothed and slightly rounded (Fig. 5-7). Nicks and points lessen the comfort and cosmetic appearance of the splint and decrease its strength.

   When cutting low-temperature materials, care should be taken to use smooth, easy cutting strokes, avoiding complete closure of the scissor blades (Fig. 5-8). A finished edge on separate splint parts that have been tubed or doubled for strength may be attained by first bonding the appropriate surfaces together and then cut-

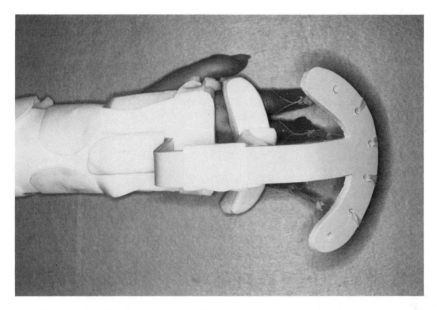

Fig. 5-6. Corners should also be rounded on accessory components such as outriggers, lumbrical bars, and finger cuffs.

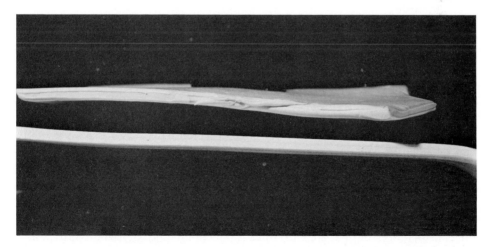

Fig. 5-7. Edge nicks and points should be smoothed into even and slightly rounded surfaces. *Top,* Poor finishing techniques; *bottom,* correctly finished edge.

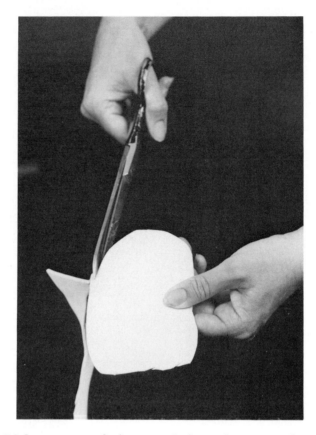

Fig. 5-8. Improper use of scissors results in rough, uneven splint edges.

ting around the edges with scissors (Fig. 5-9). Minor edge defects may be repaired by heating the edge and gently rubbing a fingertip over the defect, compressing the material into a more desirable configuration.

High-temperature materials and metals require the use of files, sandpaper, emery cloth, or steel wool for finishing edges. A novice using these materials may spend a prolonged period of time finishing edges, but with experience most splints can be finished in a maximum of 3 to 5 minutes of filing and sanding. When smoothing edges of these materials, care should be taken to avoid marring the wider, adjacent surfaces of the material (Fig. 5-10).

Analyze mechanical principles. Mechanical principles may be used to provide strength and durability to splints through adaptation of leverage systems and careful consideration of the area of force application during splint construction. Rounding inside corners increases the area of force application, diminishing the chances of material fatigue and fracture at more vulnerable corner sites. The

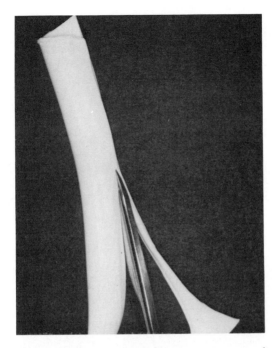

Fig. 5-9. Simultaneous cutting of bonded pieces creates a smooth single edge.

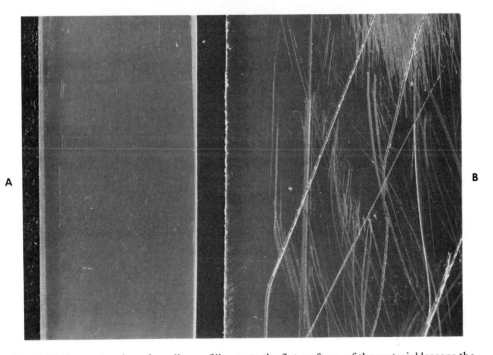

Fig. 5-10. Overextension of sanding or filing onto the flat surfaces of the material lessens the cosmetic appearance. **A,** Correct. **B,** Incorrect.

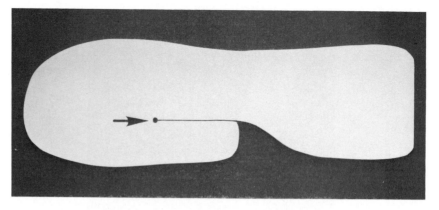

Fig. 5-11. A small hole *(arrow)* at the terminal end of an inside cut will disseminate cracking forces and increase splint durability.

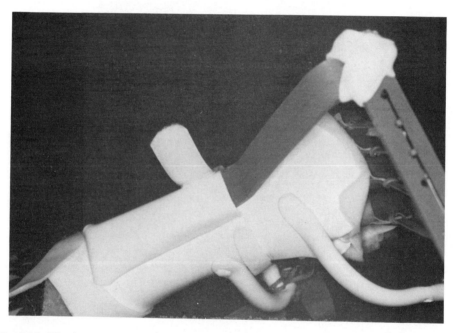

Fig. 5-12. The increased mechanical advantage (MA) afforded by a long attachment site allows for a stronger bond at the proximal end of the outrigger.

placement of a small drill hole at the end of inside cuts also disperses pressure by widening the area of force application (Fig. 5-11).

When joining splint parts, the use of one rivet will allow axial rotation, whereas two or more rivets afford a solid and stable splint joint. Providing longer sites of attachment for outriggers (Fig. 5-12) increases the durability of the bonded or riveted interface by increasing the ratio between the lengths of the resistance arm and the force arm of the outrigger.

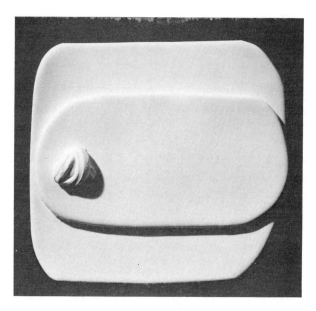

Fig. 5-13. Plastic rivets of a homologous low-temperature material provide a stable bond but may fracture with constant stress.

A careful analysis of a broken splint or splint part is an important step in determining why a splint has failed. The resulting evaluation of the force systems involved in the splint should facilitate repair and future splint preparation with technique improvement.

Stabilize joined surfaces. When a separate part must be joined to a splint, consideration of the function of the part and its requirements with regard to joint mobilization is important. An understanding of mechanical principles and the use of equipment appropriate to the material selected will ensure a more favorable result. It is important to reemphasize that, although one rivet allows motion between the joined surfaces, two or more rivets, surface bonding, or gluing results in a secure coupling of splint components. The choice of rivet type depends on the specific parts to be joined and the characteristics of the materials used (Fig. 5-13). If motion is desired in a splint, a metal rivet is more durable, and the placement of a paper spacer between the two surfaces to be joined will allow smoother rotation of the joint after the setting of the rivet and removal of the paper. Surface bonding and gluing require adherence to the techniques specific to individual materials, frequently depending on proper cleaning and heating of the contiguous surface areas for optimum results.

Finish rivets. For comfort and pleasing appearance, rivets should be flush with the material surface, particularly when they will contact the patient's skin. This may be accomplished by countersinking high-temperature materials or, in the case of the softer, low-temperature materials, by heating and molding of the rivet or the surrounding surface area. Tape or moleskin placed over an "internal" metal rivet will prevent deterioration and rusting of the rivet caused by perspiration. External rivet parts should be smooth and nonobtrusive, providing a pleasing appearance, comfort, and function.

Provide ventilation as necessary. The ventilation of a splint should be done judiciously and prudently, depending on the patient, the patient's life-style, splint configuration, and the materials employed. Splints with large skin contact areas more frequently require adaptation to improve air circulation. Ventilation holes should be small enough to prevent tissue protrusion and should be randomly positioned away from splint edges to eliminate weakening of the material (Fig. 5-14). Holes should not be situated over areas such as bony prominences that require close material contact to decrease pressure.

Low-temperature materials may be ventilated with a hand tool such as a drive punch or rotary punch (Fig. 5-15). The use of an electric drill, although suitable for high-temperature materials, is inadvisable with softer materials because it causes friction melting around the holes resulting in rough everted edges. Perforations should be made from the inside out to prepare a smoother inner splint surface, and all external hole edges should be smoothed by heating or with sandpaper, according to material type.

Commercially available perforated materials often produce poor finished products because of the preset hole pattern and the inevitable enlargement that occurs with heating and stretching during fit. Multiple, large stretched openings, rough edges, and structural weakness are the result (Fig. 5-16).

Secure padding. Padding should be used appropriately and should be anchored securely to the splint, allowing ease of splint application and removal. Increased

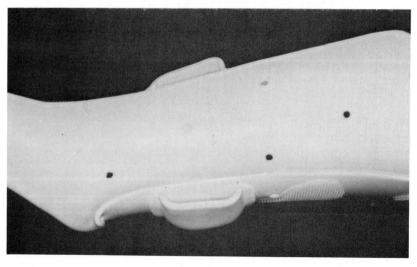

Fig. 5-14. Ventilation holes should not be placed over bony prominences, near edges, across narrow components, or in areas of high stress forces.

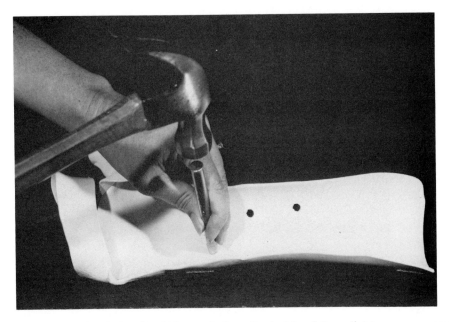

Fig. 5-15. Ventilation holes should be made from the inside of the splint to ensure a comfortable inner surface.

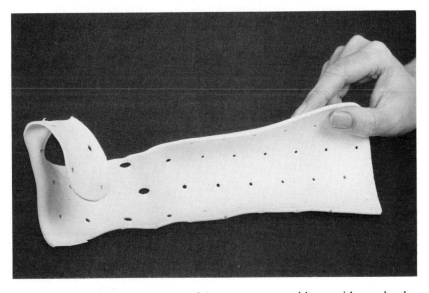

Fig. 5-16. Commercially ventilated materials may create problems with rough edges and overstretched holes.

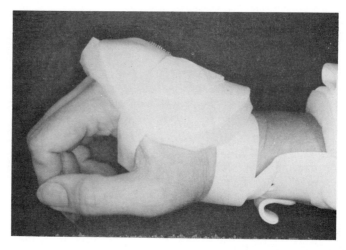

Fig. 5-17. Padding cut slightly larger than the splint part will help disseminate edge pressure.

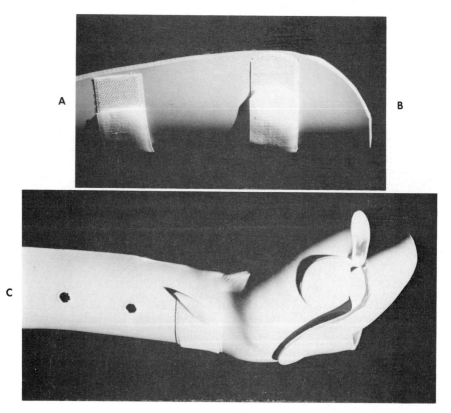

Fig. 5-18. A and **C,** With repeated closures, pointed corners on fastening strips pull away and curl, eventually resulting in detachment of the entire strip. **B,** Rounding the ends of Velcro straps and fastening strips improves appearance and increases durability.

comfort is provided when the padding material is cut slightly larger than the part to which it is to be adhered, allowing it to curl around splint edges (Fig. 5-17).

Secure straps. Straps should be strategically placed to provide splint stability on the extremity and should facilitate independent splint application and removal. They should be securely attached to the splint by riveting or gluing, and the fastening and unfastening procedure should be easily accomplished by the patient. Strap ends should be treated to prevent fraying, corners should be rounded for a more pleasing appearance and increased durability (Fig. 5-18), and overlapping soft materials should lie flat and be joined securely (Fig. 5-19), as should fastening devices such as Velcro, buckles, or snaps.

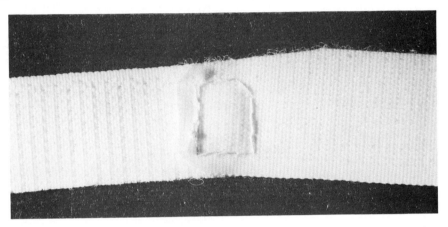

Fig. 5-19. Stitch or glue overlapping soft materials to provide a smooth durable union.

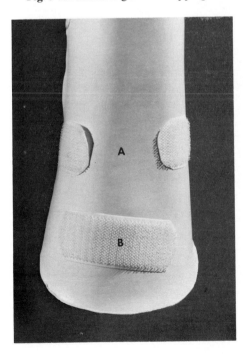

Fig. 5-20. Small button-fastening strips **(A)** that are self-adhesive or glued in place are not as durable as is a single fastening strip **(B)** that directs the unlocking forces to the center of the strip rather than to the structurally weaker edge.

When working with pressure-sensitive interlocking materials such as Velcro, the hook portion should be used sparingly because of its abrasiveness to skin and clothing. It should not comprise the length of straps but will prove durable as a fastening device when used in single lengths rather than multiple, smaller buttons (Fig. 5-20). Velcro loop straps should be long enough to provide complete coverage of the portion of hook that has been adhered to the splint, to prevent snagging and tearing of clothing, and to provide tabs that are easier to grasp (Fig. 5-21).

Straps may be adapted to facilitate use by the addition of loops or tabs (Fig. 5-22) and may be converted to adjustable straps by increasing the length and pulling through a D ring.

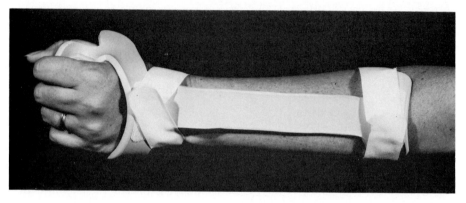

Fig. 5-21. A slight overlap of strap ends eases opening and closing and provides complete protection from hook snagging.

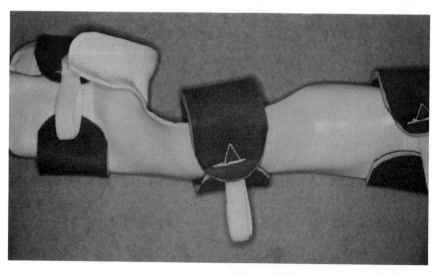

Fig. 5-22. Loops ease strap manipulation for patients with limited grasp.

SUMMARY

The principles of splint construction provide the strategic guidelines for the actual fabrication of a given splint after the design and pattern-making stages have been completed. When combined with the important principles of splint fit, the creation of a comfortably fitting, durable, and cosmetically satisfactory splint should be assured. Failure to adhere to these principles as they pertain to the sometimes trivial details of splint manufacture can often result in splint disuse because of patient discomfort, splint breakage, or, more importantly, the failure of a given splint to correctly carry out its functional assignment. To this end meticulous attention to detail is the overriding consideration; attempts to "short-cut" these construction principles to speed splint preparation will inevitably result in failure.

CHAPTER 6

Design principles and pattern construction

GENERAL PRINCIPLES OF DESIGN

Consider individual patient factors.
Consider the length of time the splint is to be used.
Strive for simplicity and pleasing appearance.
Allow for optimum function of the extremity.
Allow for optimum sensation.
Allow for efficient construction and fit.
Provide for ease of application and removal.
Consider the splint/exercise regimen.

SPECIFIC PRINCIPLES OF DESIGN

Identify key joints.
Review purpose: to augment passive motion or to substitute for active motion.
Decide whether to use static or dynamic forces.
Determine the surface for splint application.
Use mechanical principles advantageously.
Adapt for anatomic variables.
Adapt to general properties of the selected splint material.

The principles of splint design evolve from the integration of the principles of fit, mechanics, and construction. The most important consideration in splint design is the exact function expected of the splint for a specific patient. A thorough understanding of the particular problem and therapeutic goals for which a splint is required is essential to the design process. Armed with this knowledge, one can determine the ultimate configuration of the splint to be constructed. Fifteen fundamental principles must be considered in the designing of a given splint. These principles range from general to specific in nature and result in a series of decisions that will lead to the final splint design.

The principles of design may be divided into two categories. Eight general principles based on individual patient characteristics form a framework for the overall designing process of hand splints. The consideration and incorporation of these broad principles will implement the creation of a splint that is practical for both the patient and the therapist. Adherence to the remaining seven more specific principles concerned with the particular pathologic situation will help to ensure the optimum functional benefit and patient tolerance of the splint. It should be emphasized that the principles discussed in this chapter will be utilized only after there has been an appreciation of all factors unique to each patient. Decisions based on personal, technical, and medical considerations will be made. The result is often substantially different splint configurations in patients with similar therapeutic needs but different logistic or personal requirements. With experience, these decisions can be made automatically, without the need to review a detailed "checklist" of the principles listed here. Consultation with all persons involved in the rehabilitative effort must precede the actual design process and will strongly influence decisions as to splint configuration.

GENERAL PRINCIPLES OF DESIGN

The basic considerations for splint design are discussed in the following principles.

Consider individual patient factors. The individual requirements of each patient are the most influential factors in determining the ultimate size and configuration of a given splint. After the functional requirements of the splinting program are established, additional individual factors must be addressed: How much of his pathologic condition and rehabilitation program does the patient understand, and how much of the program can he intelligently accomplish for himself? How accessible is the splinting facility, and how often will he be able to return for splint adjustments or changes? To what extent will his family be able to assist him in splint application and exercises? What are the age and occupational factors?

All these factors come into careful consideration at the onset of a splinting program. Serial splints that must be changed every three to four days may present a hardship to a patient located many miles from the therapy department, and the use of an elaborately designed splint for a patient with poor motivation or an inadequate understanding of the method of splint application will almost certainly result in improper use of the splint. In addition, splints designed for use on adults may be poorly tolerated by a child, and modifications may be dictated by patient age (Fig. 6-1).

Consideration of specific circumstances such as these allow for the appropriate creation of a design which will more likely be successful because of its adaptation to the wearer's specific situation.

Consider the length of time the splint is to be used. In general, the shorter the anticipated need of the splint, the simpler its design, material type, and construction should be. An elaborately designed splint that required numerous hours to design, construct, and fit and is expected to be discarded or replaced within a few

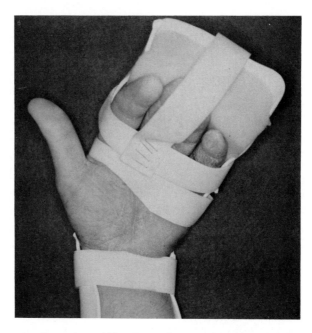

Fig. 6-1. This complex finger immobilization splint used in early passive range-of-motion of flexor tendon repairs would be contraindicated for a young child because of its ease of removal.

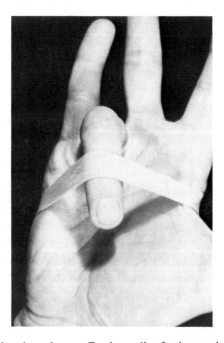

Fig. 6-2. A wide rubber band can be an effective splint for increasing proximal interphalangeal joint flexion.

days can rarely be justified to cost- and efficiency-conscious consumers, hospital administrators, and third-party participants. However, if the same splint were to be employed for three or four months, its preparation would certainly be more appropriate. Similarly, if the lifetime of the device is to be for several years or more, consultation with an orthotist may be indicated to allow for splint construction with more durable materials such as aluminum, steel, and some of the polyester resins.

Strive for simplicity and pleasing appearance. Attempts should be made to keep the overall design as simple and cosmetically pleasing as possible. At best, a hand splint is a strange-looking device, attracting attention to its wearer and further emphasizing the deformity. A poorly designed splint becomes even more obvious, lessening patient acceptance, increasing frustration, and possibly decreasing the potential for successful rehabilitation. Sometimes only a large, somewhat cumbersome splint will accomplish the desired objectives, but in many instances a simple adaptation will function equally well (Fig. 6-2). Above all, consideration for the wearer should take precedence over any impulse to design a complicated and elaborate masterpiece that may serve only as a monument to its creator!

Allow for optimum function of the extremity. The unique characteristic of the upper extremity is its ability to move freely in a wide range of motions, allowing for the successful accomplishment of a tremendous variety of daily tasks. The segments of the arm and hand function as an open kinematic chain, with each segment of the chain dependent on the segments proximal and distal to it. Compensation by normal segments when parts of the chain are limited by injury or disease will often provide for the continued functional use of the extremity. Because of this adaptive ability, splinting of the upper extremity should be carefully designed to prevent needless immobility of normal joints. For example, if digital joint limitation is caused by a capsular pathologic condition alone, the wrist may not require incorporation in the splint design. If, however, wrist position, by virtue of its effect on the osseous chain or the extrinsic musculotendinous units, directly influences distal joint motion, immobilization of the wrist may be required to obtain maximum splint efficiency. Although the mechanical purchase on a stiff joint may be enhanced by stabilization of joints proximal or distal to the joint, care should be taken to apply this concept in appropriate circumstances only. If similar results may be obtained by not stabilizing these adjacent joints, the kinetic chain will have enhanced freedom of movement.

Allow for optimum sensation. Without sensation the hand is perceptively blind and functionally limited. Because cutaneous stimuli provide feedback for activity, splint designs should leave as much of the palmar tactile surface areas free of occlusive material as possible (Fig. 6-3).

Allow for efficient construction and fit. The splint design should also allow for quick, efficient construction. With increasing concern for medical costs, long construction and fit times are for the most part inappropriate. Proper design can expedite construction and fit and decrease expense. Because each part that must be

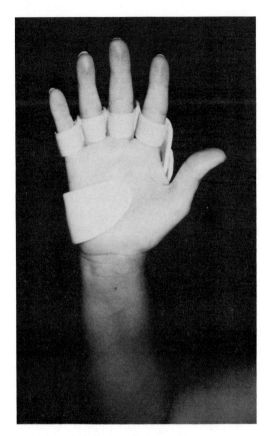

Fig. 6-3. Splints designed to leave large palmar tactile surface areas of the hand free of splint material enhance functional use. (Courtesy Joan Farrell, O.T.R., Lauderhill, Florida.)

bonded or joined will increase the construction time, the incorporation of multiple components into the main body of the splint at the design stage will result in improved efficiency. For example, providing contour at the time of designing eliminates the need for separate reinforcing strips that must be cut, formed, and bonded during the splint preparation phase. However, at times the addition of a separate piece such as a lumbrical bar may facilitate future splint adjustments without the need to modify the entire splint. Anticipation of the fit and construction factors at the design level should also eliminate much of the need for time-consuming experimentation and innovation during patient contact stages.

   Provide for ease of application and removal. Whenever possible, patients should be able to apply and remove their splints. Dependence on others for assistance may lead to frustration of both patient and family, resulting in poor wearing habits or discarding of the splint. To allow for ease of wear and removal, the splint should be designed for simple hand and forearm insertion with straps provided that may

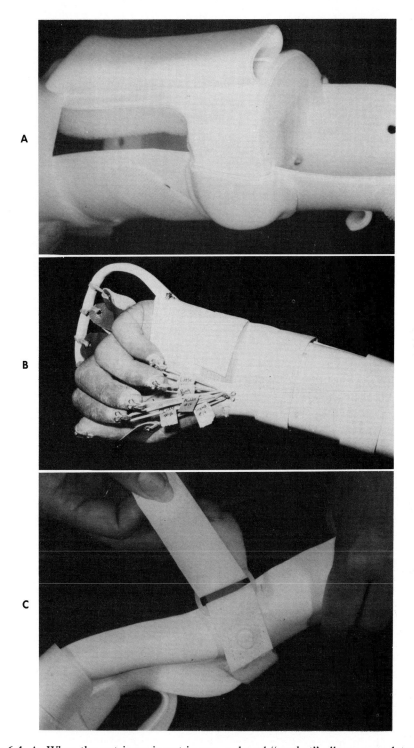

Fig. 6-4. A, When the outrigger is not in use, a dorsal "pocket" allows easy detachment from the splint. **B,** Rubber band "tags" ensure correct application of traction. **C,** Adjustable D-ring straps facilitate application and removal of bilateral complex finger and thumb immobilization splints such as resting pans or safe position splints. (**B** courtesy Joan Farrell, O.T.R., Lauderhill, Florida.)

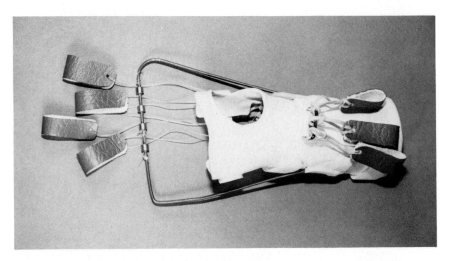

Fig. 6-5. This complex metacarpophalangeal flexion/extension splint provides two alternate passive motions in a single splint. (Courtesy K. P. MacBain, O.T.R., Vancouver, British Columbia.)

be tightened or loosened without great difficulty. Individual adaptations in the splint design, fastening devices, or method of splint application may be necessary to further facilitate patient independence (Fig. 6-4).

Consider the splint/exercise regimen. In some instances the designing of several functions into one splint may lessen patient confusion and simplify the wearing and exercise routines. For example, the amalgamation of a finger flexion/extension system into a single splint eliminates the need for a more complicated alternating two-splint routine. Efficient design considerations such as these are more clearly understood by the patient, allowing him to direct his attention more fully to his rehabilitative process (Fig. 6-5).

SPECIFIC PRINCIPLES OF DESIGN

The individual considerations, including age, intelligence, location, and lifestyle, of the particular patient are the general principles of design, with primary considerations being those of splint function, appearance, economy, and patient acceptance. The remaining seven specific principles of design stress the accomplishment of predetermined goals as defined by the unique pathologic condition:

1. What is the exact disease, injury, or deformity for which splinting is needed?
2. What are the immediate and long-term goals of the splinting regimen?
3. What is the most efficient and effective means of reaching these goals?
4. What anatomic and material variables must be considered?

These are the questions to which the specific design principles pertain.

Identify key joints. A careful evaluation of the hand with regard to existing and

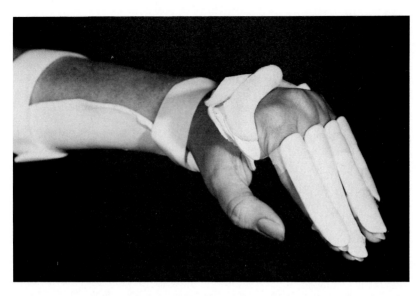

Fig. 6-6. Simple interphalangeal immobilization splints, such as these dorsal gutters, concentrate active extrinsic motion on the metacarpophalangeal joints.

potential joint mobility is perhaps the single most important consideration in determining the ultimate configuration of a hand splint. Specific recorded data obtained from active and passive range-of-motion studies will provide the examiner with an accurate assessment of motion discrepancies and allow for splint design that may effectively improve the problem areas.

After careful identification of the problem joints, decisions are made as to which joints are to be immobilized and which will receive mobilization efforts. Splints may then be designed to impart controlled forces on various digital joints to improve the passive motion and provide for a corresponding improvement in active motion.

Immobilization splinting is usually employed to allow rest or healing, to strategically position the part with the expectation of motion loss, or to gain an increased mechanical advantage at an adjacent joint. Simple gutter or close-fitting support splints are commonly used to promote healing of osseous, capsular, ligamentous, or tendon structures and to provide rest to inflamed joints and hopefully to lessen the ultimate deformity. Badly damaged joints with no expectation of functional salvage may be splinted to allow stiffening in the most favorable position.

A static splint may also be used on one or more joints to augment the mechanical forces at another joint by allowing an increase or decrease of tension on musculotendinous units. Maximum benefit of a dynamic splint may be obtained by immobilizing joints proximal or occasionally distal to the injured or diseased joint (Fig. 6-6). When loss of motion is a problem at only one joint of a given digital ray, dynamic traction to the entire segment will result in the dissipation of force

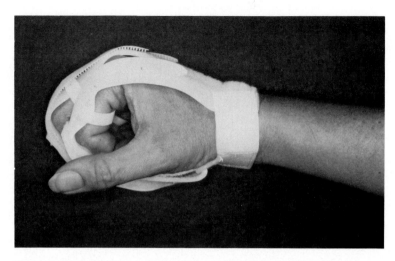

Fig. 6-7. This type of simple finger flexion splint employs inelastic traction to increase passive flexion of the digital joints.

on the normal joints with little effect on the problem area. When all joints of the segments are equally impaired, the necessity of immobilizing proximal or distal joints is less important (Fig. 6-7).

When dealing with a particularly difficult situation in which numerous joints are involved, it is sometimes helpful to mark the joints with a water-soluble felt-tip pen, using an easily identifiable code for the joints to be mobilized and those to be immobilized (Fig. 6-8). This method or other graphic techniques that allow clear visualization of the splinting objectives are extremely important to correct splint design.

Review purpose: to augment passive motion or to substitute for active motion. After identifying key joints, one must review the specific functional objective of a given splint. Is it desirable to increase or to maintain the passive range of motion or to substitute for absent active motion? Substitution splints frequently provide control of function and may be fabricated of more durable, less adjustable materials because of their expected length of use. An example of a substitution splint is the use of a cock-up splint to provide wrist extension in radial nerve paralysis or a piano wire splint (Fig. 6-9) to restore a flexion restraint at the metacarpophalangeal joints in ulnar nerve paralysis. To be effective, a substitution splint requires full passive joint motion. If full joint excursion is not present, a different splint is first required to decrease the existing deformity. Splints designed to augment passive range of motion are often temporary and should be easily adaptable because of configurative changes as the arc of motion increases. The more pliable plastic materials should be employed for these splints.

It is imperative that the designer of the proposed splint clearly understand the reason for the application of the splint and adapt the design accordingly.

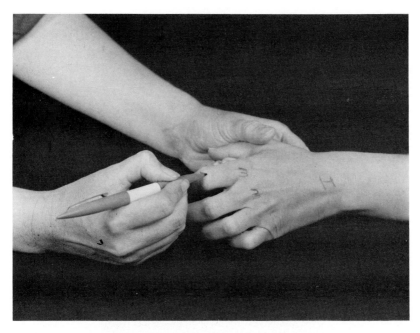

Fig. 6-8. In complicated cases, graphic identification of joints to be mobilized and immobilized may aid in splint design.

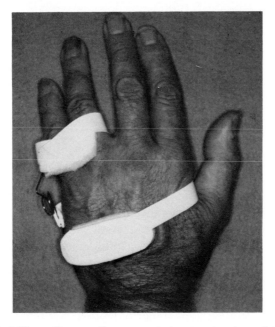

Fig. 6-9. A modified Wynn Parry splint prevents hyperextension of the fourth and fifth metacarpophalangeal joints in ulnar nerve paralysis.

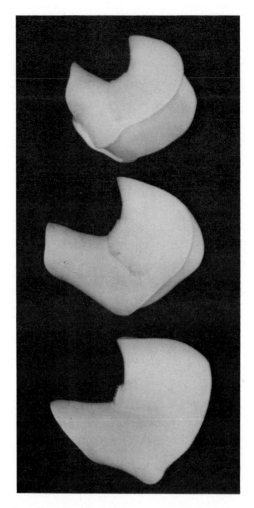

Fig. 6-10. Static thumb web spacers may be used serially to increase carpometacarpal joint passive motion.

Decide whether to employ static or dynamic forces. Concomitant with the recognition of splint purposes and the identification of key joints is the decision regarding whether the proposed splint should function statically or dynamically. Most static splints immobilize joints and generally are more simple in concept and design than are dynamic splints. Static splints affect only joints that they cross, and their success is primarily dependent on usage of favorable mechanical advantage and the recognition of kinematic and anatomic variables. Static splints may also be used serially to enhance passive range of motion of a joint (Fig. 6-10), providing a form of "inelastic traction."

Dynamic splints are often more complicated in design and necessitate the use

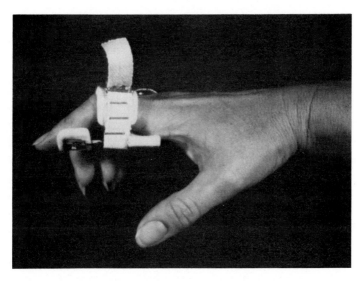

Fig. 6-11. Inelastic traction is often more efficient than elastic traction in decreasing interphalangeal flexion stiffness of 30 degrees or less.

of specific mechanical principles to achieve optimal functional results. The choice between elastic and inelastic traction for mobilizing joints frequently depends on the joint to be mobilized and its specific range of motion. For example, inelastic traction in the form of serial web spacers will often produce better results in increasing motion at the thumb carpometacarpal joint than will conventional dynamic splints using elastic traction. This has also proved true for increasing extension of a proximal interphalangeal joint whose extension deficit is 30 degrees or less (Fig. 6-11). Decisions at this level in the design will result in major changes in the final configuration of the splint.

Determine the surface for splint application. The decision as to what surface or surfaces of the hand or forearm the splint is to be applied is the next step in the progression through the hierarchy of design principles. This decision is influenced by the interrelationships of anatomic and mechanical factors. Although pressure is usually better tolerated on the volar surface of the extremity, one must be aware of the fact that this side makes the greatest contribution to function and sensation. A dynamic extension splint is mechanically more efficient when based dorsally, and a volar splint best enhances dynamic flexion forces. Ulnar deviation of the wrist may be statically controlled from either the ulnar or radial surface, but if ulnar deviation is to be dynamically achieved, the splint should be based on the ulnar aspect of the forearm.

Use mechanical principles advantageously. The employment of mechanical principles will add detail and dimension to the development of the hand splint. These principles determine the length and width of the splint, regulate splint position, define the angles of attachment of the traction devices, and may help identify additional splint components. Failure to consider and adapt to these principles may result in an ineffective or uncomfortable splint that may have otherwise been designed appropriately.

Adapt for anatomic variables. Individual anatomic variables, abnormal structures, or defects may also influence the design of the splint and are important in the choice of surface on which the proposed splint will be based. A skin graft over the dorsum of the forearm may preclude dorsal construction, as would the presence of significant dorsal synovial swelling over the carpus. A prominent radial styloid process is a frequent problem in volarly applied splints that incorporate the wrist.

Adapt to general properties of the selected splint material. Adaptation of design to incorporate the properties of available materials is also an important consideration in the fabrication of hand splints. Many of the low-temperature materials require splint designs that provide strength and support through increased contour of the material to the hand. A bar type of splint constructed from these materials would be an inappropriate design choice because of the inherent weakness of the material. Technical difficulties in splint fabrication must also be considered to avoid unfortunate or ineffectual results when working with a particular material. If the material has a high cohesive or bonding factor, a circumferential design may increase fit problems when overlapping ends bond together unexpectedly, and the choice of a rigid material for a design whose success depends on a close fit may predispose frustration and failure.

The general principles of design form the basic framework of knowledge on which any hand splint must be based, whereas the specific principles, altered by individual patient variables and functional requirements, will influence the final configuration of the splint. The experienced therapist does not employ these principles one by one in checklist fashion but considers them simultaneously, adding, eliminating, and supplementing them with innovation and creativity. The challenge is to create a splint that not only meets the functional objectives but is acceptable and well tolerated by the patient.

PATTERNS

The transition from the cognitive design process to the actual construction of tangible splint patterns is facilitated by the progression through the hierarchy of design principles. Once the design process has been traversed, the construction of a workable pattern becomes simplified. Assembly and connection of the various splint parts may then be carried out until the ultimate configuration of the splint becomes apparent. This allows alterations of shape and size to be governed by individual specifications of the extremity being splinted before actual fabrication of splint materials has commenced.

In the pattern stage, simple splints with uncomplicated objectives will allow for rather routine application of design principles, whereas in the presence of unu-

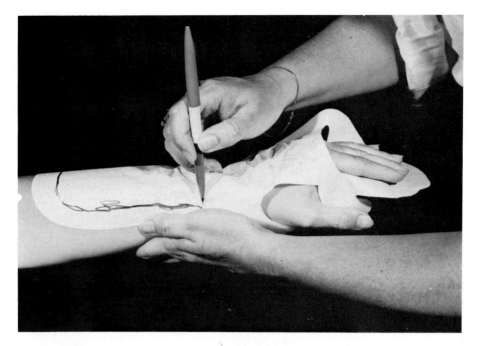

Fig. 6-12. A commercial pattern must be adapted to the variations of the individual hand before it is used.

sually difficult problems a more innovative approach will be required. Nevertheless, a progression through the prescribed design stages will facilitate a more efficient, organized thought process from which practical variations can be made.

The rigid use of standard, commercially available patterns is not recommended because it may result in the preparation of a splint without the appropriate adaptation necessary to accommodate individual anatomic variations. With experience comes the knowledge of where and how to incorporate changes in these dye patterns, and the potential hazards are diminished considerably (Fig. 6-12). All patterns, whether individually constructed or adapted from a commercial design, should be fitted and checked on the patient before construction of the splint begins, since a poorly conceived or fitted pattern will almost always lead to frustration and failure during the subsequent stages of construction, fit, and use.

Splint pattern fabrication

The fabrication of splint patterns may be defined according to the construction methods employed: (1) the combining of individual splint parts, (2) the outlining of the total splint configuration, or (3) the taking of specific measurements to form a general pattern shape.

All patterns, like the splints they represent, consist of individual parts that, when combined, form a whole. For the beginner or for the experienced individual attempting to translate a difficult splint design into pattern form, taping and combining cut-out paper splint parts on the patient's extremity may facilitate pattern construction (Fig. 6-13). An alternate technique of pattern fabrication, the drawing of an outline of a splint, is more efficient when dealing with familiar, uncomplicated splint designs. The uncut pattern material is first applied to the extremity, and the configuration of the proposed splint outlined according to anatomic

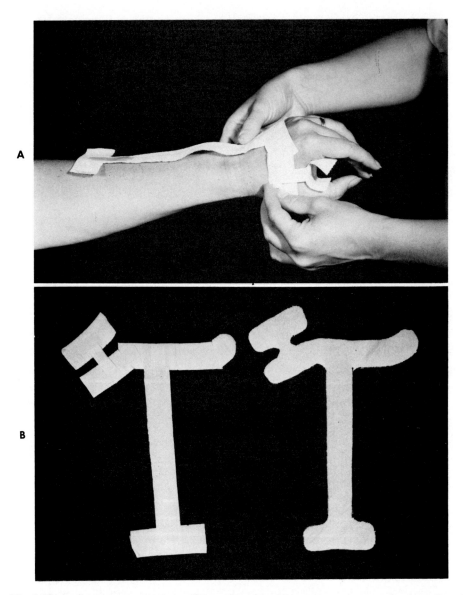

Fig. 6-13. A, A component pattern allows piece-by-piece pattern construction based on the specific requirements of the hand being splinted. **B,** Once the basic form is established, the outside configuration of the pattern is smoothed and refined.

landmarks and mechanical considerations (Fig. 6-14). These two methods of pattern construction may be effectively combined to blend the efficiency of the outline method with the specificity of the parts technique (Fig. 6-15). The third method of pattern construction is appropriate only when a stretchable splinting material is to be used. This less exacting technique of pattern preparation results in a pattern that bears little resemblance to the finished splint. Length and width

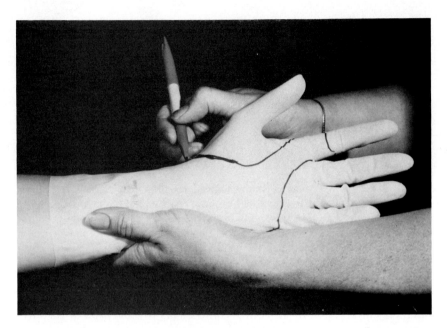

Fig. 6-14. Outline pattern construction is more expedient for uncomplicated designs.

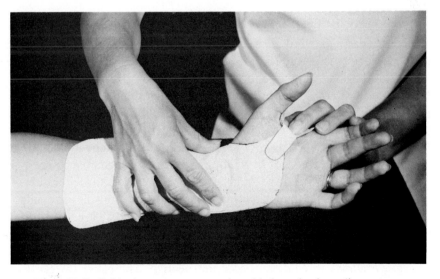

Fig. 6-15. Individual components may be added to a basic outline pattern.

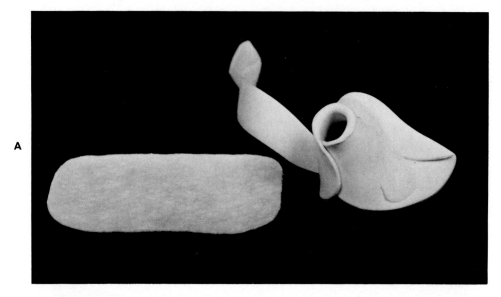

A

Fig. 6-16. **A,** As seen in this short opponens pattern design by Kay Carl, O.T.R., Indianapolis, Indiana, measurement patterns often bear little resemblance to the final splint configuration. **B,** The length between dorsal and volar wrist flexion creases through the first web space is the pattern length. **C,** The length from the index proximal interphalangeal joint to the thumb interphalangeal joint equals the width.

measurements are frequently the only requirements for this type of pattern construction because the splint material is stretched, molded, and trimmed during the fitting phase of fabrication (Fig. 6-16).

Pattern materials and equipment

Although pattern materials are of seemingly infinite variety, they possess some common properties. They should be readily available, inexpensive, flexible, clean, and allow for marking, taping, and cutting. Examples are paper towels, typing paper, cloth, light cardboard, cellophane, plastic wrap, clear plastic bags, and surgical gloves. The choice of pattern material may be influenced by the splint design, pathologic condition of the extremity, material accessibility, or environmental factors. A pattern for a splint requiring contour would be difficult to make from light cardboard because of its mildly rigid properties, whereas a bar type of splint pattern out of plastic wrap would be flimsy and could allow alteration of the splint form during transfer to the final splint material. Paper towels are available in most medical offices and therapy departments and are flexible enough to allow contouring. Cellophane, plastic bags, and plastic wrap provide the unique property of transparency, giving full visibility to underlying anatomic structures, and a surgical glove allows three-dimensional perspective. The paper towels that are

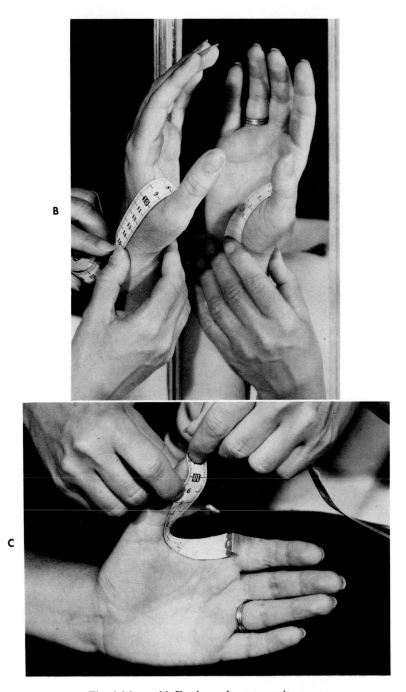

Fig. 6-16, cont'd. For legend see opposite page.

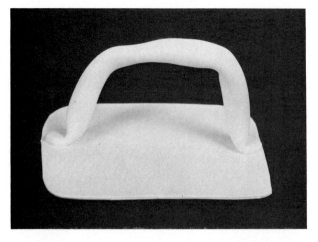

Fig. 6-17. A positioning device may be used to support a paralyzed hand during pattern construction.

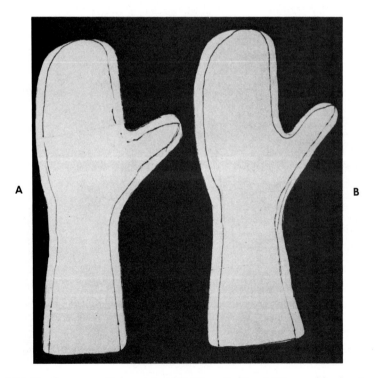

Fig. 6-18. Resting pan pattern made with (**A**) and without (**B**) a positioning device.

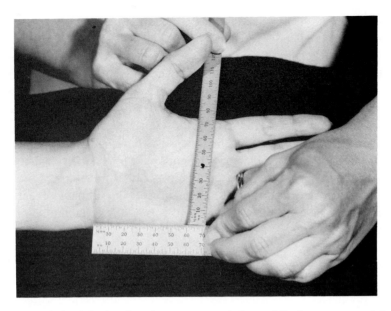

Fig. 6-19. The width of the hand at the metacarpophalangeal flexion crease and the length from the wrist flexion crease to the metacarpophalangeal flexion crease on the ulnar aspect of the palm are the two most important measurements to take when attempting to locate a similar-sized hand for pattern construction.

provided with sterile surgical gloves also make excellent pattern materials when working in isolation conditions.

Positioning devices (Fig. 6-17) have been advocated in some circumstances when making a single plane pattern proves to be difficult. These devices allow the various segments of the extremity to be placed in the desired position, theoretically making tracings more accurate. In our experience, however, the final configurations of patterns made with and without a positioning device are similar enough that the addition of an extraneous piece of equipment is usually unwarranted (Fig. 6-18).

If it appears that the amount of hand movement required to construct a pattern will be poorly tolerated by the patient, a pattern may be traced from the opposite, unaffected hand, allowing for individual variations such as edema or amputation. This pattern should then be reversed and checked for fit on the injured extremity. If the pathologic condition disallows pattern construction on either extremity, longitudinal and horizontal measurements may be taken (Fig. 6-19), and a hand of similar size located on which a pattern may be made.

SUMMARY

It is important that a complete understanding of the principles of splint design precede the actual preparation of any device intended to protect or improve hand function. Reckless, disorganized fabrication of splints, although sometimes more expedient, will not only fail to meet the functional goals of the splint itself, but may be poorly fitted, mechanically incorrect, or may actually contribute to deformity.

Although it may initially seem that the review of a large number of general and specific principles of splint design is redundant and time consuming, it will soon become clear that the principles can be approached in a logical, sequential fashion and will, with repetition, actually provide for simpler, more efficient splint preparation. Consideration of the desired splint purpose, based on the individual problem presented by the patient, is obviously the important first step in a splint construction. Sequential review of the general principles of design, followed by the application of the more specific principles, will allow for the ultimate preparation of a splint that will best meet the desired objectives of the rehabilitation team and, most importantly, be satisfactory for the optimum functional result of the patient.

CHAPTER 7

Positive and negative molds

A negative mold provides the external frame or shell for a positive reproduction of the hand in plaster, dental acrylic, or similar material. The negative mold is prepared directly on the patient's hand. After removal, it is filled with a liquid material that, through an endogenous heat process, dries and hardens. When this material is completely solid, the negative mold is peeled away, leaving a positive duplication of the hand. This positive mold may then be used in the fabrication of splints and in the education of persons involved in wearing or making hand splints. The intent of this chapter is to acquaint the reader with the basic purposes of negative/positive molds and to briefly describe the construction process of these molds with two differing materials: plaster and dental acrylic.

Because early splint materials were often too caustic or too hot to be placed directly on a patient's skin, positive molds were indispensable in providing inert replicas on which splints could be fitted without harm to the patient. When necessary, the construction of negative/positive molds added considerably to fabrication time, and, because they produced rigid duplications of normally mobile structures, the splints shaped to the molds frequently required further refinement to accommodate active hands, again adding to the total fabrication time. With the advent of low-temperature plastics that allow warm splint materials to be fitted directly to the patient, the need to produce positive molds for splint fabrication has almost disappeared. Considering the efficient splint fabrication currently possible because of the technologic advances in materials, it would be impracticable to insist on making a negative/positive mold system for every patient requiring a hand splint. There are, however, specific instances when their production is indicated.

The use of positive molds can be invaluable in teaching patients, students, and other professionals (Fig. 7-1). For example, studying a splint without the corresponding anatomic landmarks can confuse and mislead even the most experienced clinician, to say nothing of its effect on an apprehensive patient who has never encountered such a device. When the splint is placed on a positive mold of a hand, however, familiar points of reference are readily apparent, allowing the patient or student to direct full attention to the instructions or explanation being given, instead of groping for spatial orientation. Serial positive molds can also provide a

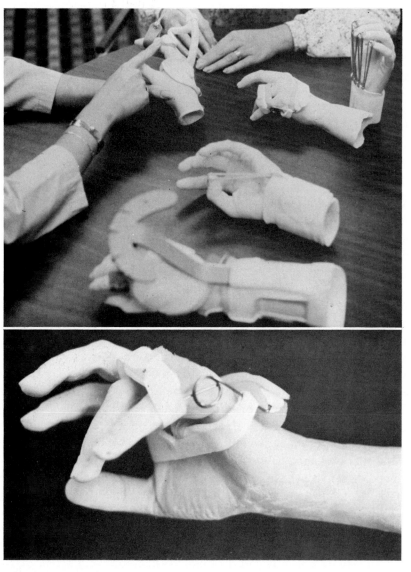

Fig. 7-1. Positive molds used as visual aids may be of considerable assistance in the education of patients or students.

permanent three-dimensional record of postural changes in the hand as a result of therapeutic or surgical intervention or through a pathologic process occurring over a period of time (Fig. 7-2). In addition to providing permanent records of the changes in deformity in a given hand, these serial molds can be of considerable assistance in general patient counseling and teaching situations. There are also specific occasions when a positive mold may be helpful because of unusual patient circumstances, either environmental or medical. For instance, patients needing periodic splint replacement for whom the hand clinic is inaccessible or inconven-

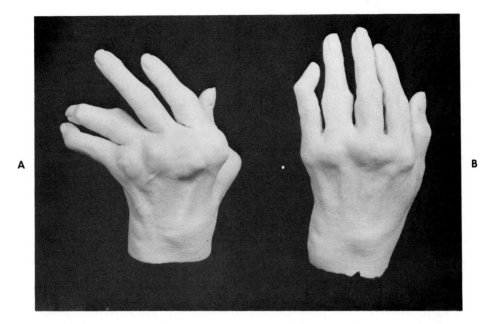

A   B

Fig. 7-2. Molds may provide a permanent record of postural changes in the hand, as does this set of preoperative (**A**) and postoperative (**B**) molds.

ient because of transportation problems can benefit considerably by having permanent duplications of their hands available at the clinic, allowing additional splint fabrication without their presence.

Although medical circumstances necessitating construction of positive molds are rare, they can and do occur. Overly anxious, hypersensitive, or hyperactive individuals comprise the majority of problem patients in this area, often requiring some means of anesthesia for the fabrication of the negative mold. A final situation requiring the preparation of a negative/positive system of molds may be found in cases in which high-temperature plastics, caustic materials, or metal must be used for splint construction. Because metal wears or fatiques plastic, resulting in unstable, malaligned splint components, a metal base splint may be preferable. The use of a positive mold during the construction and fitting processes of a metal splint frees the patient from involvement in tedious hours of splint fabrication.

As previously mentioned, two methods of constructing molds will be described in this chapter. Although the fundamental concepts are identical with these two methods, the use of differing materials produces positive molds with heterogeneous physical properties. The choice of material is dependent on the ultimate use intended for the positive mold. Although both techniques require similar construction times, plaster is considerably less expensive but produces a more fragile, less detailed finished product that is sufficient for splint fabrication but lacks the durability needed for teaching models which are handled and used daily. The more expensive dental acrylic molds are durable, and, if made correctly, reproduce the minute surface detail of the original hand (Fig. 7-3). It is important to note that the chemical reaction producing the endogenous heat process for curing the dental acrylic is toxic to the respiratory system, requiring a well-ventilated room for dissipation of the resultant fumes.

To employ time efficiently and reduce the ultimate clutter, all materials and equipment for the preparation of hand molds should be collected and arranged before initiating work on the negative mold. Both patient and work area should have protective coverings, including drop cloths on the floor. If the patient is unable to independently maintain the hand posture required, an assistant should be present to help.

PLASTER MOLDS
General considerations

Plaster cures through endogenous heat created by a catalytic reaction between water and crystalized gypsum. The strength of plaster is proportionate to the ratio of plaster of Paris and water, and its curing time can, to some extent, be regulated by adjusting the water temperature. An increased temperature externally augments the catalytic heat response and decreases the curing time. Plaster-impregnated bandage is available in a range of approximate setting times and should be selected according to the specific task and the expertise of the clinician. Wet layers of plaster bandage should be worked until the plaster layers are integrated and smooth. During the 20- to 30-minute curing time necessary for most plaster

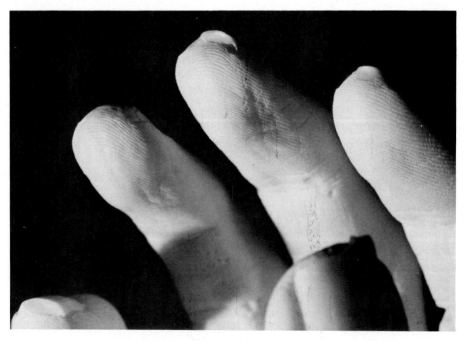

Fig. 7-3. Fingerprints and skin creases are exactingly reproduced in this positive mold of dental acrylic.

bandage molds, adjustments should be minimal because disruption of the plaster molecules at this stage may cause weakness in the mold.

Liquid plaster should be mixed to the consistency of heavy cream, avoiding whipping motions that induce air bubbles into the mixture. The molds into which liquid plaster is poured should be rotated and gently tapped to release air bubbles trapped by the contours of the mold.

Fabrication of a negative plaster mold

  Materials

  Apron, smock

  Newspaper, plastic sheeting

  Pan of warm water

  Bandage scissors

  Petroleum jelly

  Paper towels

  Three rolls of fast-curing 2-inch plaster bandage

  Procedure

    1. Cover patient and work area with protective garments or materials.

    2. Precut plaster bandage strips according to length of intended mold and size of the hand and forearm. Following are measurements for a forearm and hand mold on an adult patient:

       a. Twelve to fifteen 14-inch lengths (includes 2-inch distal overlap) for forearm/hand

Text continued on p. 165.

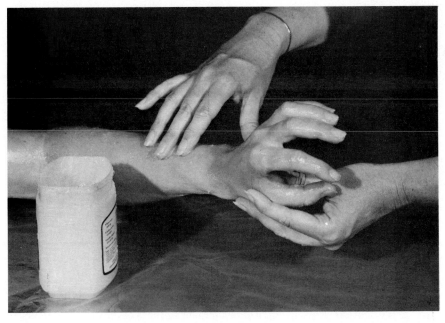

Fig. 7-4. Hair should be thoroughly covered with petroleum jelly to prevent adherence to the inner surfaces of the negative mold.

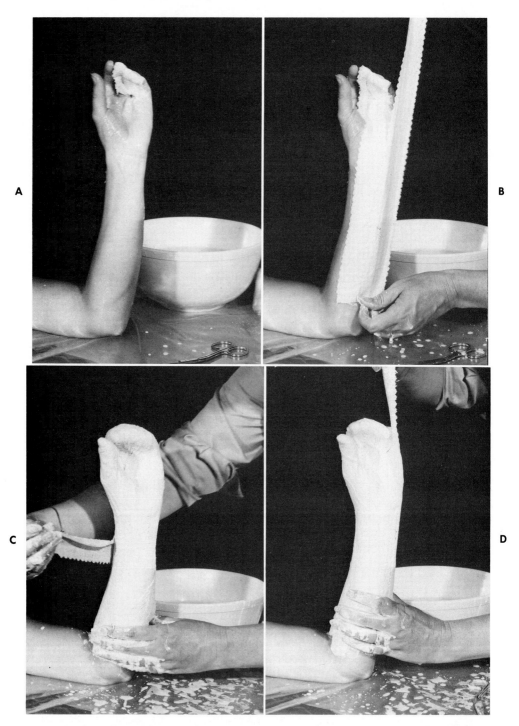

Fig. 7-5. A to **C,** Plaster strips are applied to alternate surfaces of the hand and thumb until, **D,** a thickness of three layers is reached.

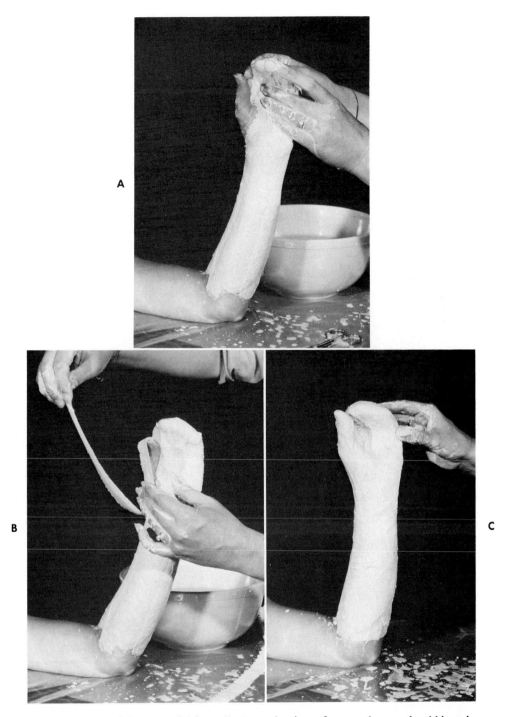

Fig. 7-6. Because of the potential for collapse at the time of removal, care should be taken to reinforce the thumb, first web space, and fingers.

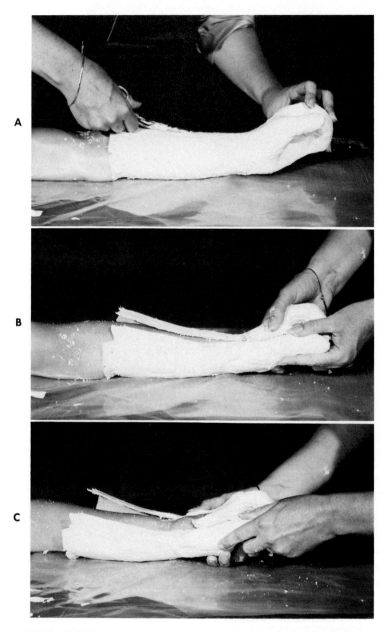

Fig. 7-7. A, The radial Y-shaped opening allows extraction of the hand from the plaster negative. Because of pressure from the scissors on underlying tissue, the course of the cut should run slightly dorsal to the prominences of the head of the radius and first metacarpal and slightly volar to the lateral aspect of the second metacarpal. **B to E,** Once the cut is complete, the negative mold is removed from the hand by gently pulling distally.

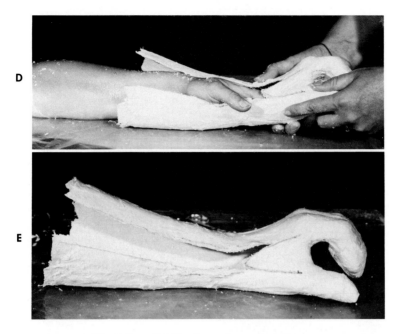

D

E

Fig. 7-7, cont'd. For legend see opposite page.

    b. Several ½-inch widths 8 inches long for reinforcement of thumb, first web space, and fingers
    c. One 18- to 24-inch length for final spiraling wrap
3. Evenly coat patient's arm and hand with petroleum jelly, taking care to cover dorsal hair (Fig. 7-4).
4. Position fingers, wrist, and thumb.
5. Roll strips, and as needed dip into water, gently wringing to remove excess water.
6. Apply wet strips longitudinally to forearm and hand, alternating dorsally and volarly. The 2-inch additional length of each strip is brought around fingertips and run in a proximal direction to provide overlapping of strip ends. Work around forearm with overlapping strips until two or three layers have been worked together (Fig. 7-5).
7. Narrower bandage strips are preferable when working on thumb and reinforcing first web space and fingers (Fig. 7-6).
8. The final strip should be spiraled around extremity, providing circumferential stability.
9. Allow plaster to set approximately 10 to 15 minutes.
10. Loosen negative mold by having patient pronate and supinate forearm.
11. Cut mold with bandage scissors to allow extraction of hand. Cut should be in the shape of an elongated Y following radial aspect of forearm and first and second metacarpals (Fig. 7-7).

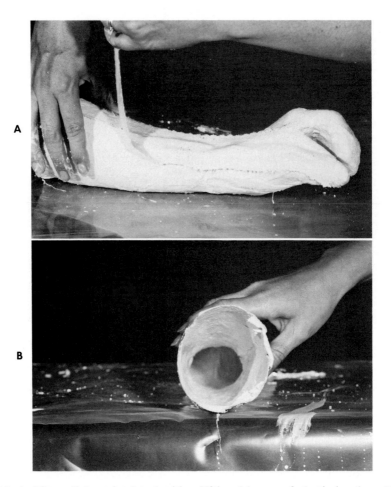

Fig. 7-8. A, The radial cut is closed with additional layers of plastic bandage. **B,** Visual examination of the internal surfaces of the mold by holding it to a light source will reveal weak areas in the layers of plaster.

12. Remove negative mold by pulling gently in a distal direction.
13. Close the radial cut and externally reinforce weak areas of negative mold with additional strips (Fig. 7-8).

Fabrication of a positive plaster mold
  Materials
  Apron, smock
  Newspapers, plastic sheeting
  Plaster of Paris
  Two basins
  Water
  Separator (1 part kerosene, 1 part liquid soap)
  Pencil
  Dowel rod or pipe (optional)

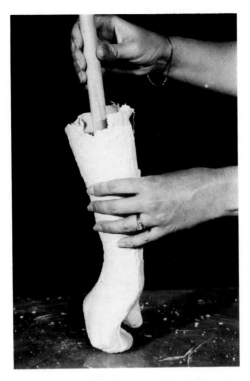

Fig. 7-9. A dowel rod incorporated into the positive mold at the time of pouring allows the finished mold to be secured in a vise.

Procedure

1. Cover work area with protective material.
2. Hold negative mold over basin, and pour approximately one cup of separator into mold. Coat all internal surfaces by rotating mold. Pour remaining separator in mold back into original container.
3. Mix plaster and water to consistency of heavy cream. The amount depends on size of negative mold.
4. Pour small amount of wet plaster into negative mold, rotating and shaking mold to allow plaster to flow into the more distal crevices.
5. Fill mold with plaster, and continue to rotate and shake mold gently to dislodge air bubbles.
6. If a dowel rod is to be included in the positive mold (Fig. 7-9), it should be inserted into the wet plaster and held until plaster is solid enough to support it.
7. When plaster maintains an impression, inscribe patient's initials and date to facilitate mold identification.
8. When plaster is completely solid and cool to the touch, gently peel negative mold away from positive mold. During this process, special care should be taken when working on thumb or isolated fingers because of the ease with which they break.

9. Finish the positive mold by lightly smoothing surface irregularities with fine sandpaper.

SILICONE RUBBER AND DENTAL ACRYLIC MOLDS
General considerations

It is important to be aware that, because of noxious fumes produced by catalytic reaction, the fabrication of molds from Silicone rubber or dental acrylic must be carried out in a well-ventilated area. In contrast to the rigid plaster bandage negative mold, a Silicone rubber negative mold is slightly flexible, allowing for easier extraction of the patient's hand from the mold. Both Silicone rubber and the dental acrylic require the addition of a separate catalyst to create the endogenous heat necessary for the conversion from a liquid to solid state. As with the plaster technique, care should be taken to minimize the amount of air bubbles in the liquid materials during the mixing and pouring stages by avoiding whipping motions and by rotating and tapping the filled negative mold. The curing process may be accelerated by increasing the ratio of catalyst to base material. Care should be taken to not cause a too-rapid setting time, which results in insufficient time to apply the material or to pour it into a mold. Because the positive and negative materials are not homogeneous, the application of a separator to the internal surfaces of the negative mold is not necessary.

Fabrication of a silicone rubber negative mold
Materials
Apron, smock
Newspapers, plastic sheeting
Dow Corning 310 RTV Silicone rubber
Dow Corning RTV Catalyst No. 1 or No. 4
Petroleum jelly
Paper towels
Wax paper
9-inch paper cups
Tongue depressors
Procedure
1. Protect patient and work area with appropriate coverings.
2. Place sheets of wax paper over immediate work area.
3. Coat hand and arm lightly with petroleum jelly. Too much jelly will decrease the final amount of surface detail. Be certain to adequately cover hair.
4. Pour catalyst into 9-inch cup, rotating to evenly coat inner surfaces. Pour excess back into bottle.
5. Fill cup to 2 inches from top with Silicone rubber, and mix thoroughly with tongue depressor.
6. Position patient's thumb, fingers, and wrist.

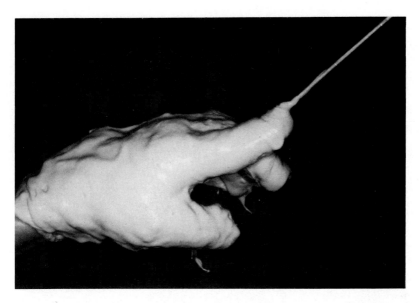

Fig. 7-10. To ensure adequate coverage, careful attention should be directed to the web spaces and adjacent finger surfaces.

7. Pour mixture slowly over patient's forearm and hand as patient gradually pronates and supinates extremity. Scrape excess material from wax paper and reapply to hand. Cover all areas of hand and forearm with substance (Fig. 7-10).
8. Once extremity is covered, maintain hand posture until curing process is complete (approximately 15 to 30 minutes).
9. Begin hand removal process by having patient pronate and supinate forearm and hand.
10. If negative mold includes forearm, it may be necessary to make small cut in negative mold at radial wrist level to allow hand to be pulled out of mold, depending on individual hand size and configuration.
11. Remove mold by gently pulling in distal direction (Fig. 7-11).
12. Externally repair any cuts or tears in negative mold with tape or Silicone rubber.

Fabrication of a dental acrylic positive mold
  Materials
  Apron, smock
  Newspapers, plastic sheeting
  Syborn Kerr Formatray powder
  Dow Corning Catalyst M (stannous octoate)
  9-inch paper cups
  Tongue depressor

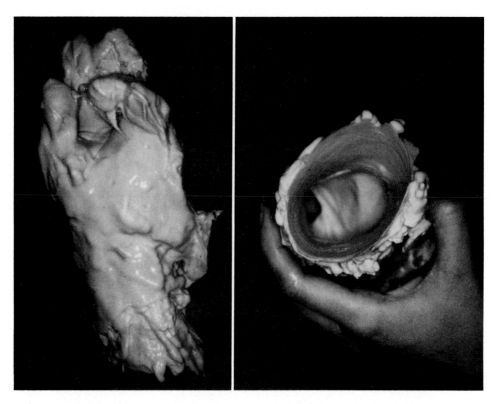

Fig. 7-11. The patient may assist in removal of the negative mold by gently pronating and supinating the hand and wiggling the fingers.

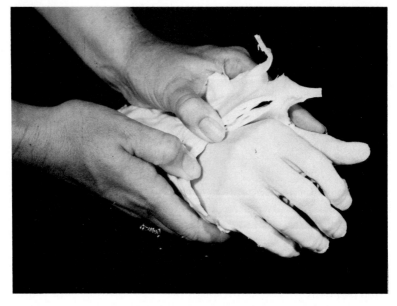

Fig. 7-12. Because the materials are heterogeneous, the negative mold is easily peeled away from the positive without the need for an intervening separator substance.

Procedure
1. Protect work area with appropriate covering.
2. Pour dental acrylic powder into cup to 4- to 5-inch level.
3. Add catalyst and mix. Material should be consistency of heavy cream.
4. Pour into negative mold, gently shaking and rotating mold to free bubbles trapped by mold contours.
5. Mix second batch of dental acrylic, if needed, and pour in similar manner.
6. Allow acrylic to fully cure (material becomes very warm and then cools).
7. Peel Silicone rubber negative mold away from positive mold (Fig. 7-12).
8. Finish by sanding or filing surface irregularities from positive mold.

SUMMARY

Although negative/positive molds are not used as they formerly were, a definite place remains for the technique in certain clinical situations. In addition, accurate hand reproductions created by these methods may be of considerable value in teaching clinicians and educating patients, as well as providing a permanent record of a particular hand or changes in its deformity.

CHAPTER 8

Splints acting on the wrist

The osseous anatomy of the wrist consists of the distal radius and ulna and eight carpal bones. The wrist is classified as a condylar diarthrosis with a wide range of motion resulting from its many small internal joints and intrinsic stability provided by a complex ligamentous arrangement. As the most proximal segment in the intercalated chain of hand joints, the wrist is the key to function at the more distal joint levels. Because the wrist is vulnerable to a wide assortment of injuries and diseases, it is subject to acute or secondary patterns of deformity, instability, or collapse, that can prove markedly detrimental to hand performance.

The combined motion of the wrist results in hand positioning in the sagittal, coronal, and transverse planes. The collective carpal bones form the anteriorly concave proximal transverse arch, whose functional position directly influences the kinetic interaction of structures composing the longitudinal arch. It appears that the traditional concept of the wrist carpus as two transverse four-bone rows is a substantial oversimplification of its complex dynamic motion patterns. Taleisnik (1978), in refining the work of Navarro, defines the carpal scaphoid as the lateral or mobile column of the wrist, with the triquetrum serving as the medial or rotation column and the remaining six bones comprising the central or flexion-extension column. Taleisnik points out that the anatomic positioning of the wrist ligaments, particularly on the volar side, permits these intricate columnar movements and provides the best rationale for understanding the dynamic anatomy of the wrist, its function, and its behavior during injury.

It is generally agreed that radial deviation and flexion of the wrist occur primarily at the midcarpal joint, whereas ulnar deviation and extension are predominantly a radiocarpal motion. Direct or adjacent trauma, particularly when accompanied by crushing or prolonged edema, may result in fibrotic changes in the tightly articulated wrist joints with a resulting limitation of motion. The obligatory immobilization of fracture, tendon, or ligament injuries in this area increases the possibility of motion loss. Conversely, ligamentous rupture or attenuation secondary to inflammatory disease processes may result in wrist instability and collapse patterns that may compromise digital performance to an even greater extent than that produced by wrist stiffening.

Because the wrist serves as the key joint to distal hand function, influencing both digital strength and dexterity, it is important that great consideration be given to proper joint positioning and protection, as well as the attainment and maintenance of a satisfactory range of motion. A program that integrates splinting and exercise often provides the essential elements in the preservation of wrist function.

It is also important that the effect of wrist position be thoroughly considered in the preparation of any hand splint. Wrist dorsiflexion tightens extrinsic flexor tendons and permits the synergistic wrist extension–strong finger flexion function employed in power grasp. Wrist volar flexion tightens the long extrinsic extensor tendons, allowing the hand to open automatically, while greatly reducing digit flexion efficiency. Splints designed either to relax or protect extensor tendons or to promote active digital flexion should be designed to incorporate the extended wrist, whereas active digital extension or flexor tendon healing is enhanced by splinting the wrist in a flexed attitude. Understanding of these kinetic mechanisms and their careful application can often augment healing and motion programs in the hand.

The purpose of this chapter is to discuss splinting of the wrist with regard to anatomic, kinesiologic, and mechanical factors. There are six basic reasons for splinting a wrist:

1. To protect injured or repaired structures.
2. To prevent deformity.
3. To decrease pain.
4. To enhance distal function.
5. To correct deformity.
6. To increase the purchase on more distal joints.

It is much more common to use wrist splints for immobilization purposes. With the limited exception of splints designed to correct wrist deformation, all wrist splints in the preceding list require immobilization techniques.

SIMPLE WRIST SPLINTS

To control articular motion, simple wrist splints affect motion of the multiple carpal joints in a similar manner. They may be used to mobilize or to immobilize.

Immobilization

As has been mentioned, simple wrist immobilization splints are important in allowing healing of injured structures intrinsic to the distal forearm and wrist. Depending on the purpose of application, these splints may be fitted to affect motion in either or both the sagittal and coronal planes.

The most commonly used simple wrist immobilization splint is the dorsiflexion or cock-up splint, which, except in special circumstances, positions the wrist in approximately 30 degrees of extension to allow maximal composite hand function. Radial and ulnar deviation bars are frequently employed to prevent coronal movement of the hand (Fig. 8-1). For optimum mechanical advantage, the forearm trough should be two thirds the length of the forearm and half its thickness.

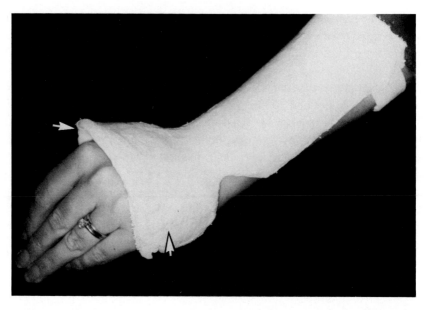

Fig. 8-1. The use of deviation bars *(arrows)* prevents lateral and medial motion of the hand in this plaster splint designed to immobilize the wrist and inhibit metacarpophalangeal flexion of the ring and small fingers.

The metacarpal bar should allow full metacarpophalangeal flexion and extension, and, if possible, straps should be placed at the far distal and proximal ends of the splint and directly over the wrist axis of rotation. Care should be taken to diminish pressure over bony prominences such as the ulnar styloid process and the head of the radius.

Mobilization

Mobilizing the stiffened wrist by splinting is a most difficult assignment. Certainly no externally applied splinting device can selectively differentiate its force application to the radiocarpal or midcarpal joints. When columnar wrist motion patterns are considered, the problem of mobilizing pathologically fibrosed wrist joints becomes even more difficult. Nonetheless, carefully prepared dynamic splints that attempt to gently loosen immobile carpal articulations without damaging uninjured ligamentous structures may on some occasions prove beneficial.

Simple wrist mobilization splints may be fitted to produce wrist flexion, extension, or deviation and are usually constructed as a single unit or as two pieces connected by a traction device or joints (Fig. 8-2). Both types should allow continuous 90-degree angle of pull to be employed through the use of appropriate length outriggers. If the wrist is passively mobile, an outrigger may not be required. The wrist bar is absent in the two-piece splint and hinged in the single-

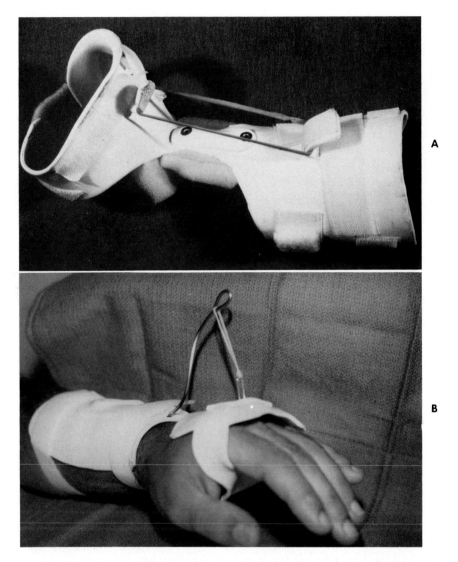

Fig. 8-2. A simple wrist mobilization splint may be designed as a single unit (**A**) or as two pieces (**B**). Depending on the position and mobility of the wrist, use of an outrigger to provide a 90-degree angle of pull to the metacarpals enhances the mechanical function of the splint. (**B** courtesy Cynthia Philips, O.T.R., Boston, Massachusetts.)

piece splint (Fig. 8-3). To reduce pressure, the longitudinal length of the metacarpal bar should be as long as possible without inhibiting wrist motion proximally and metacarpophalangeal motion distally. It should also maintain the distal transverse metacarpal arch. Thumb motion should be preserved, and the forearm trough should be two thirds the length of the forearm and, if using low-temperature plastic, half its thickness. An elbow cuff may be necessary to prevent distal

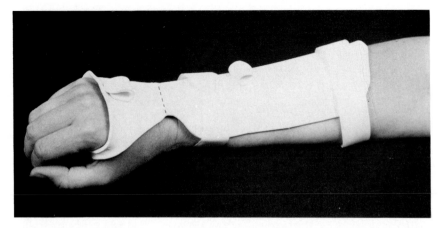

Fig. 8-3. A hinged wrist bar must be aligned *(broken line)* with corresponding wrist creases to permit uninhibited motion.

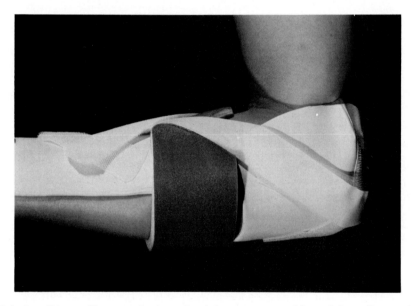

Fig. 8-4. An elbow cuff may assist in maintaining correct position of the splint on the extremity. (This patient was unable to tolerate a triceps cuff.)

migration of the forearm trough (Fig. 8-4). Because of the magnitude of the forces involved in mobilizing a wrist, careful attention should be directed to underlying cutaneous surfaces. The splint should be removed for skin inspection a minimum of every hour during the initial wearing phase. Padding is usually necessary at the distal end of the forearm trough and along the length of the metacarpal bar. It is not unusual for a wrist mobilization splint to produce transient median nerve

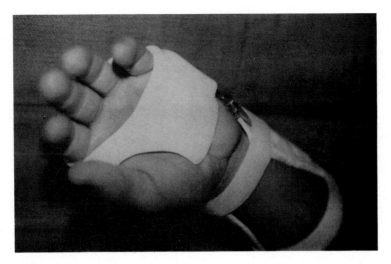

Fig. 8-5. A jointed wrist splint is often used in the postoperative care of a patient who has undergone a wrist arthroplasty procedure. (Courtesy Cynthia Philips, O.T.R., Boston, Massachusetts.)

compression with paresthesias in the distribution of the nerve. If a patient complains of numbness in the fingers from wearing the splint, it should be removed and adjusted. If the numbness returns when the adjusted splint is reapplied, the splint should be discontinued.

Some wrist mobilization splints allow motion in one plane but inhibit motion in another, usually through the use of jointed hand and forearm pieces (Fig. 8-5). In fitting this type of splint, it is imperative to match the rotational axis of the splint with the anatomic joint axis. Malalignment of the two joints may inhibit motion and cause friction abrasions to underlying skin.

COMPLEX WRIST MOBILIZATION SPLINTS

In the presence of passively supple joints, tendon adhesions may inhibit simultaneous passive flexion or extension of both the wrist and digital joints secondary to a tenodesis phenomenon. To increase tendon excursion and convert the tenodesis effect, a splint must be designed to either immobilize the wrist and mobilize the fingers or mobilize the wrist and immobilize the fingers. Either method will enhance the mechanical focus of the dynamic traction. Although both types of splints would be categorized as complex, the mechanical emphasis of each is different, as are their descriptive classifications: complex finger mobilization splint and complex wrist mobilization splint, respectively.

In a complex wrist mobilization splint the posture of the wrist and the direction of the traction are dictated by whether flexor or extensor tendon excursion is limited. When flexor tendon adhesions are present, a finger pan may be used to immobilize the fingers in extension, while dynamic extension traction is applied to

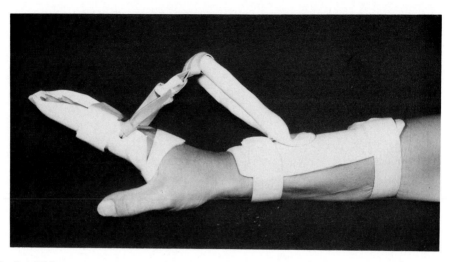

Fig. 8-6. This complex wrist extension splint may be used to decrease the tenodesing effect of extrinsic flexor tendon adhesions.

the wrist (Fig. 8-6). If extrinsic extensor adhesions limit simultaneous wrist and finger flexion, the fingers may be immobilized in a flexed attitude, and gentle flexion traction applied to the wrist. For optimum rotational effect, the traction assist for either splint should pull at a 90-degree angle to the metacarpals and should also be perpendicular to the center of the sagittal axis of rotation of the wrist. The metacarpal bar should support the distal transverse metacarpal arch and, in the case of the complex wrist flexion splint, should allow full metacarpophalangeal flexion. The forearm trough should be of sufficient length and width to provide good mechanical advantage and strength.

As previously mentioned, efforts to mobilize digital joints may be compromised by the position the wrist is allowed to assume. The tenodesis effect of wrist extensors on digital flexors is an important consideration in the design of complex finger splints with wrist immobilization components. Although the wrist is included as an adjunctive measure, the primary purpose of these complex finger mobilization or immobilization splints is directed toward influencing digital status. For this reason further discussion of these types of splints will be included in the chapter dealing with splints acting on the fingers.

SUMMARY

The integrity of the wrist joint with its complex anatomic and motion arrangements has been established as the "key" to hand function. It is uniquely vulnerable to a variety of injury and disease processes that can result in pain, stiffness, or instability, which may greatly operate against normal hand function at all levels. The management of these wrist maladies may be substantially enhanced by proper splinting with objectives ranging from pain relief and protection to prevention and correction of deformity. In addition, wrist splinting can be used to negate or augment long extrinsic tenodesis functions in the management of digital pathologic conditions. It is therefore imperative that careful consideration be directed toward the anatomic, kinesiologic, and functional effects of any splint created to traverse this important joint.

CHAPTER 9

Splints acting on the fingers

The purpose of this chapter is to examine the concepts of splinting the fingers. Governed by anatomic, kinesiologic, and mechanical variables, these splints must also adhere to the principles of design, fit, and construction. The most common reasons for applying finger splints are the correction or prevention of deformity and the protection of injured or repaired structures. Finger splinting may also be used to decrease pain or enhance grasp and release patterns.

The functional capacity of the fingers is dependent on the integrated mobility of its four proximally unified, distally independent articulated rays. These triarticular units function as diverging open kinematic chains whose four segments provide a progressive summation of motion in the sagittal and coronal planes. The mobility afforded by the fourth and fifth carpometacarpal joints also provides an element of motion in the transverse plane to the ring and small fingers, allowing volar and radial approximation of the ulnar border of the hand. Longitudinally each successive joint adds an increment of sagittal mobility until at its maximal limit the cumulative palmar flexion possible per digit is approximately 280 degrees. The condylar metacarpal joints also allow some passive rotation in addition to flexion, extension, abduction, and adduction of the fingers.

The effect of a single articular restriction or the loss of a distal segment on composite hand function is lessened by the presence of multiple normally functioning joints that allow continued hand use. However, as the number of stiffened joints or lost segments increases, the compensatory ability of the hand becomes progressively compromised.

In addition to supple joints, muscles of adequate strength with adhesion-free tendinous excursions are required to provide the necessary power and control to produce highly integrated digital motion responses. In their normal state the fingers represent an equilibrium of intrinsic and extrinsic forces that, in conjunction with the thumb, are capable of functional patterns ranging from delicate prehension to powerful grasp.

Because digital effectiveness is dependent on mobility, it is important to achieve and maintain adequate motion early in the rehabilitation process. Splinting and exercise programs should be designed to prevent the development of articular and musculotendinous limitations. In the presence of established deformity, emphasis should be placed on restoring lost motion. Programs should acknowledge the structural peculiarities at each joint level and be designed accordingly. The metacarpophalangeal joints of the fingers have a propensity for becoming stiff in extension; the proximal interphalangeal joints more often become stiff in flexion.

Sensation also plays an important role in finger usage. Impaired digital sensation diminishes the ability of the hand to distinguish texture and pressure variables. This inability to adequately receive, relay, or interpret sensory impulses from the hand will severely limit composite hand function. Splints whose designs encourage hand use should not encumber the palmar surfaces of the fingers, particularly at distal, more tactilely important levels.

IMMOBILIZATION SPLINTS

Finger immobilization splints may be used to promote healing, control early postoperative motion, or enhance functional use. These splints may involve one or more joints and, depending on the specific requirements, may be fitted dorsally, volarly, laterally, or circumferentially. Care should be taken to maintain correct ligamentous stress at each joint incorporated in the splint and to permit full motion of the uninvolved joints. Maximum three-point mechanical advantage may be ensured by straps placed over key joints and each end of the splint (Fig. 9-1). Because of their long narrow configurations, finger immobilization splints should be contoured to half the phalangeal segmental thickness to augment material

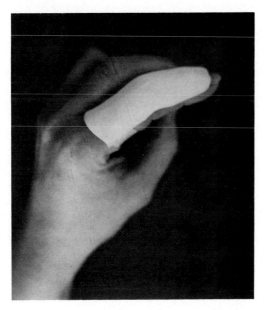

Fig. 9-1. Tape is often used to secure an immobilization or blocking splint to the finger.

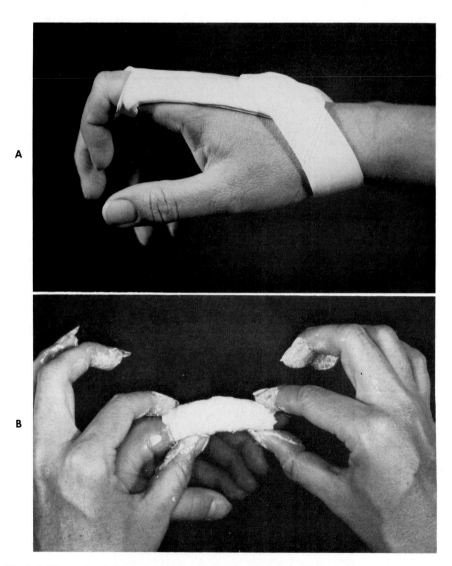

Fig. 9-2. These simple immobilization splints prevent articular motion (**A**) at the metacarpo-phalangeal joint, (**B**) at the proximal interphalangeal joint, and (**C**) at the distal interphalangeal joint, as well as (**D**) of the entire ray (dorsal and volar views). (**D** courtesy Joan Farrell, O.T.R., Lauderhill, Florida.)

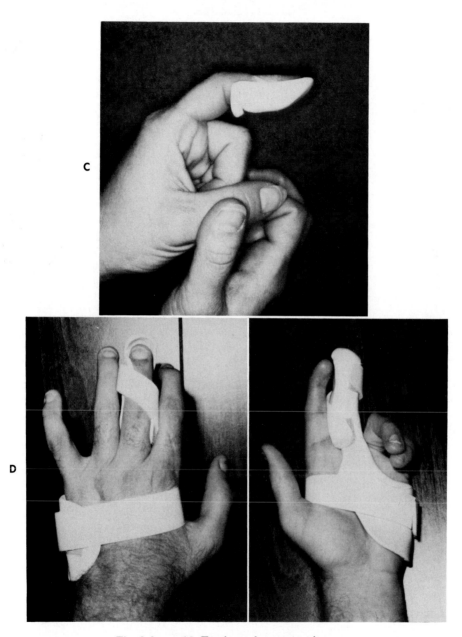

Fig. 9-2, cont'd. For legend see opposite page.

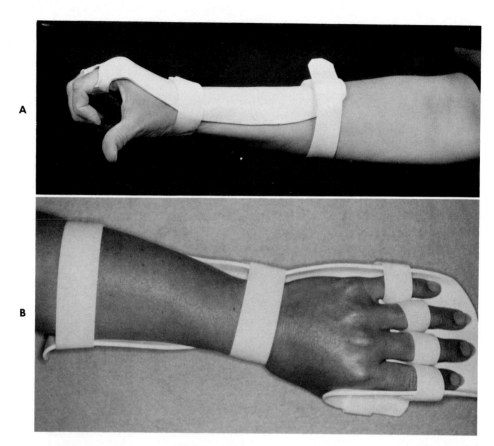

Fig. 9-3. Complex finger immobilization splints may partially inhibit motion of a longitudinal ray (**A**) or completely immobilize the fingers (**B**).

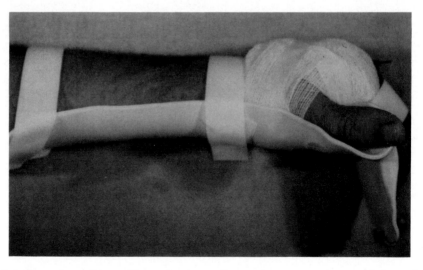

Fig. 9-4. The safe position splint maintains optimum stress on metacarpophalangeal and interphalangeal collateral ligaments.

strength, and splint length should be extended as far distally and proximally as possible without inhibiting motion of uninvolved adjacent joints.

Finger immobilization splints may be categorized as simple or complex, depending on whether the wrist is incorporated or allowed unrestricted motion. Whereas simple splints prevent articular motion (Fig. 9-2), complex finger immobilization splints influence extrinsic musculotendinous units (Fig. 9-3) by means of adjunctive wrist positioning. Wrist position may be used to increase or decrease the amount of tension on these musculotendenous units through alteration of the tenodesis effect. The forearm trough of a complex immobilization splint should be half the thickness of the forearm and two thirds its length.

It should be stressed that, for immobilization of finger joints which have not undergone surgical repair, the preferred or "safe" position for the metacarpophalangeal joints is usually considered to be 70 to 90 degrees of flexion, and a 5- to 10-degree flexion posture is best for the interphalangeal joints (Fig. 9-4). These attitudes considerably decrease the potential for ligamentous contractures and the consequent limitation of articular motion.

MOBILIZATION SPLINTS
Metacarpophalangeal level

The metacarpophalangeal joints of the index, long, ring, and small fingers are of the condyloid type in which the rounded metacarpal head fits into a small concavity at the base of the proximal phalanx. The ligamentous arrangement at each joint consists of two collateral ligaments and one volar ligament that allow anteroposterior and mediolateral motion in addition to a slight amount of passive phalangeal rotation. The collateral ligaments are slack when the joint is in extension and taut when the joint is flexed. Pathologic conditions involving the metacarpophalangeal joints of the fingers frequently result in periarticular stiffness and eventually contracture in a position of extension or hyperextension. This type of deformity in a protracted state is extremely difficult to correct through conservative means. It is important to anticipate this problem and make appropriate efforts to maintain adequate length of the metacarpophalangeal collateral ligaments through preventive flexion splinting and exercise programs that emphasize full metacarpophalangeal joint flexion.

Splinting for mobilization of a metacarpophalangeal joint should incorporate a 90-degree rotational force on the distal aspect of the proximal phalanx, which is also perpendicular to the axis of rotation in the desired plane of the involved joint. If a perpendicular pull is not achieved, unequal force will be applied to the periarticular ligaments, which may cause stretching and result in ulnar or radial deviation of the digit. To allow full flexion, the volar metacarpal bar of a metacarpophalangeal flexion splint should not extend beyond the distal palmar flexion crease. If distal migration of the splint limits metacarpophalangeal motion, an elbow cuff or diagonal splint straps may be added to further stabilize the splint on the extremity. The choice between a simple (Fig. 9-5) or complex (Fig. 9-6) splint

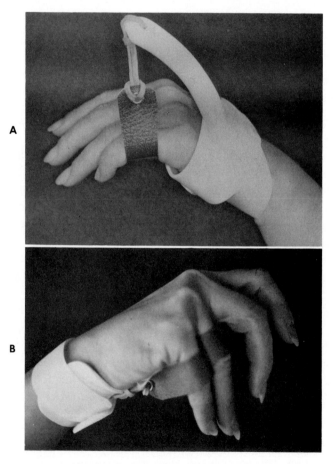

Fig. 9-5. Simple metacarpophalangeal splints may augment (**A**) extension, (**B**) flexion, (**C**) abduction, (**D**) adduction, or (**E**) rotation.

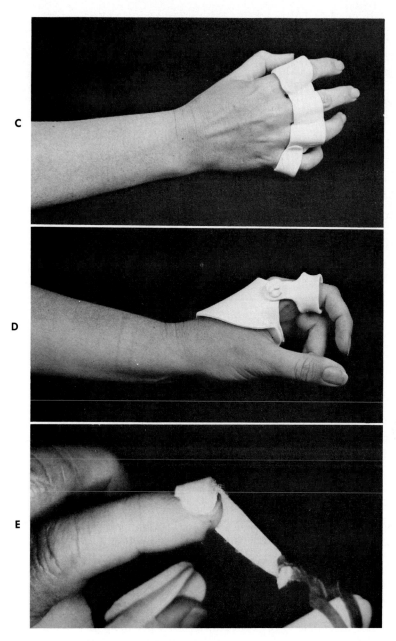

Fig. 9-5, cont'd. For legend see opposite page.

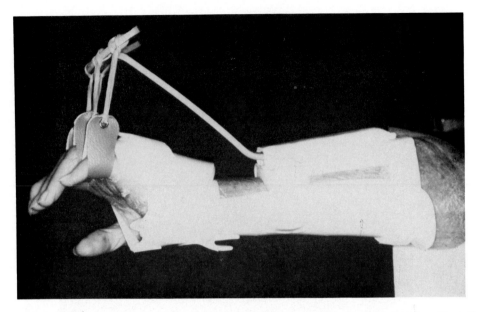

Fig. 9-6. Complex metacarpophalangeal splints immobilize the wrist to control the effect of extrinsic musculotendinous adhesions or myostatic contracture on more distal digital joints.

design depends on the presence or absence of extrinsic adhesions producing a tenodesis effect or poor habitual posturing of the wrist.

Proximal interphalangeal level

The interphalangeal joints of the fingers are true hinge joints and allow motion in only the sagittal plane. The ligamentous structure of these joints is similar to that of the metacarpophalangeal joints in that there are two collateral ligaments and one volar plate ligament per joint. However, the interphalangeal joints differ from the metacarpophalangeal joints in that the articular surfaces of the interphalangeal joints travel in the same arc throughout their full range and produce a constant tension on the collateral ligaments regardless of joint position. These joints, unlike the metacarpophalangeal joints, have a tendency to develop flexion contractures, although they may become contracted in extension as well.

Splinting for interphalangeal joint mobilization requires that the angle of approach of the rotational force be 90 degrees to the middle phalanx. This force should also be perpendicular to the axis of joint rotation to create equal stress on the collateral ligaments (Fig. 9-7). Because the proximal interphalangeal joint is the intermediate joint of the three digital articulations, splints that influence it often must affect the joints proximal and distal to it. If all the joints within the ray possess similar degrees of mobility, and if wrist position does not affect digital motion, a simple splint design may be appropriate (Fig. 9-8). However, if discrep-

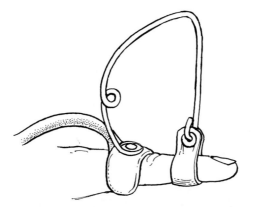

Fig. 9-7. For maximum benefit of traction, the angle of approach should be 90 degrees to the proximal phalanx and perpendicular to the axis of rotation.

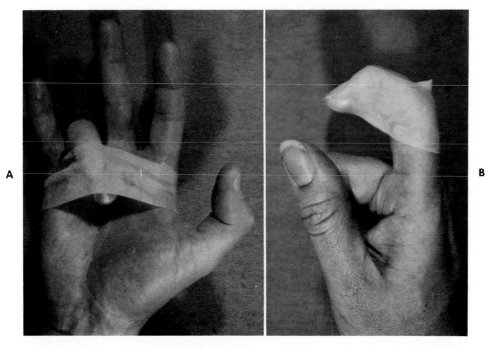

A B

Fig. 9-8. Simple proximal interphalangeal mobilization splints may affect the proximal interphalangeal joint alone or influence other joints within the ray in a similar manner (**A** and **B**).

ancies exist in the relative mobility of the successive joints within the digital ray, measures should be taken to control the more mobile joint and allow traction to be concentrated on the stiffer joint. Compound splint designs may provide concomitant stabilization of a segment and mobilization of another within the same longitudinal ray (Fig. 9-9). When wrist patterns are poor, or when decreased extrinsic musculotendinous amplitude creates a tenodesing of finger joints, wrist immobilization may be used to control the extrinsic influence at the digital level (Fig. 9-10). A forearm trough and wrist bar may be added to a simple or compound splint design to create an appropriate complex splint. When multiple joints of a ray are incorporated within a splint, there is little room for error because the multiple

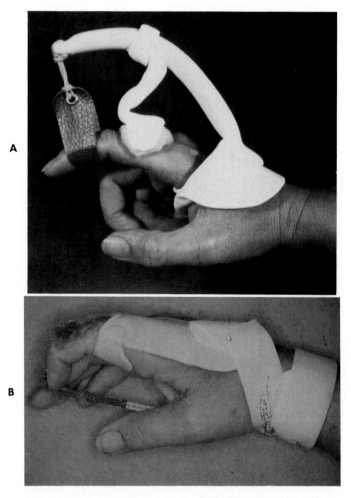

Fig. 9-9. These compound proximal interphalangeal mobilization splints stabilize the proximal phalanx and focus the extension (**A**) or flexion (**B**) traction force on the proximal interphalangeal joint.

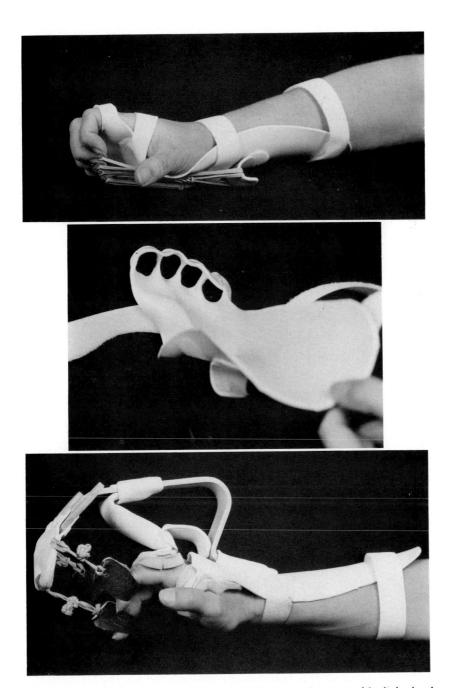

Fig. 9-10. Complex proximal interphalangeal mobilization splints resemble their simple and compound counterparts distally but immobilize the wrist proximally.

lever arms involved tend to accentuate deformity. Care should be taken to ensure that the mobilizing force influences each joint correctly.

Experience has shown that splints such as the safety pin or joint jack are more effective in correcting flexion deformities that measure approximately 35 degrees or less. A joint whose fixed flexion is greater than 35 degrees responds more readily to a short dorsal outrigger with lumbrical bar or to serial cylinder casts. Experience has also shown that consecutive serial casting of extremely stiff joints results in better passive motion than was achieved with elastic traction on the same joints.

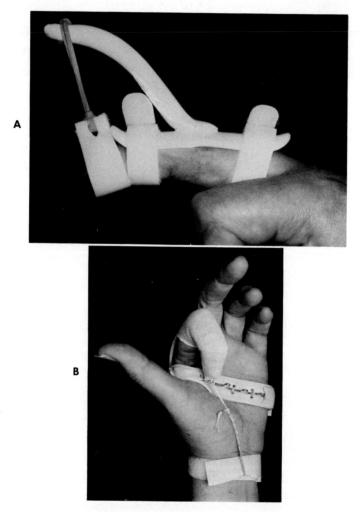

Fig. 9-11. Distal interphalangeal mobilization splints may produce less favorable results than do their proximal interphalangeal joint counterparts. **A,** Compound distal interphalangeal extension splint. **B,** Simple distal interphalangeal flexion splint. (**B** from Hollis, L. I.: Innovative splinting ideas. In Hunter, J. M., et al., editors: Rehabilitation of the hand, St. Louis, 1978, The C. V. Mosby Co.)

Distal interphalangeal level

Because the distal interphalangeal joints are also hinge articulations, mechanical principles similar to those of the proximal interphalangeal joints are applicable. From a practical point of view, however, the small area of purchase provided by the distal phalanx makes elaborate dynamic traction techniques less applicable for stiffness at this joint. Three-point pressure splints such as static gutters, cylinder casts, safety pin splints, or joint jacks may prove most effective in correcting flexion deformities, and simple straps or rubber bands may best overcome extension stiffness (Fig. 9-11).

SUMMARY

Pericapsular fibrosis resulting in stiffening of the metacarpophalangeal or interphalangeal joints of the fingers represents the most common disabling problem following hand injury, disease, or surgery. The use of preventive splints that immobilize joints in positions least favorable to stiffness or mobilizing splints designed to overcome existing contracture are important components of the equipment of those involved in the hand rehabilitative process. A sound knowledge of factors contributing to the pathologic condition at a given joint is required in making decisions as to the type and design of a given digital splint. As with splints at other levels, decisions with regard to splint purpose and realistic expectations must be made and explained to the patient with careful monitoring of splint performance leading to appropriate alterations in the specific management of digital deformities.

CHAPTER 10

Splints acting on the thumb

The importance of the thumb in almost all aspects of hand function cannot be overstated. The presence of an opposable thumb gives the human species a manual dexterity that is unparalleled in lower animal forms. Insurance companies assess a 40% functional loss to a hand that is missing the thumb, and the real loss may be substantially greater. Because of the tremendous disability resulting from thumb loss, hand surgeons have long strived to develop techniques to salvage or restore thumb function such as that lost as a result of congenital absence, traumatic amputation, disease, or injury.

The functional requirements of the thumb differ substantially from those of the other four digits. Thumb stability, for example, is much more important than mobility, and a thumb unit with basilar joint motion alone may permit adequate function despite fused distal joints. Even a completely immobile first metacarpal can serve as a stable post for prehension with the mobile adjacent digits if it is in the correct position. In addition to stability, it is important that the thumb unit retain sufficient length for pinch and grasp functions and sensation of at least a protective grade without pain and hypersensitivity. The maintenance of proper thumb position, therefore, is of extreme importance, and splints that correct thumb deformities, establish and maintain an adequate first web space, and help mobilize stiffened thumb joints are among the most important discussed in this book.

The thumb is a multiarticular, open kinematic chain that moves through three planes and combinations thereof. The distal segment of the chain is allowed a high degree of freedom of movement as the result of the summation of the participating joints. This arrangement helps minimize the disabling effect of the restriction or loss of motion at any of the individual joints as the result of trauma or disease.

Splinting may be employed to immobilize the thumb or thenar segments to allow healing, control early postoperative motion, or enhance functional use. Inflammatory conditions and soft tissue injuries of thenar structures often require splint immobilization. Postoperative immobilization between exercise periods effectively limits use while allowing early motion, and static positioning of a paralyzed or partially paralyzed thumb aids in the prevention of deformity while permitting continued functional use.

Because optimal effectiveness of the thumb is dependent on its mobility, preservation or restoration of motion of the three joints is an important part of the re-

194

habilitation process. Splinting and active range-of-motion exercises, combined with purposeful activity, are the cornerstones of this process. Maximum passive range of motion of the involved joints must be acquired and maintained before a corresponding active range of motion can be achieved or before surgical procedures may be attempted. Splinting is generally accepted as the most effective non-surgical means for achieving an improved passive range of thumb motion.

Regardless of the intent of splint application, the basic principles of mechanics, design, construction, and fit must be implemented to create a splint that meets the requirements of the specific situation. The purpose of this chapter is to discuss splinting techniques as they relate to the thumb.

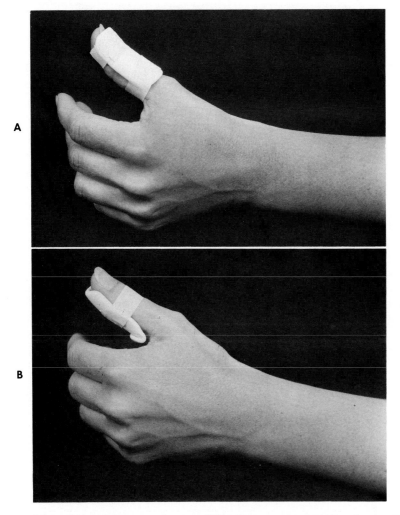

Fig. 10-1. Although the placement of straps differs between dorsal (**A**) and volar (**B**) simple thumb immobilization splints, the mechanical function of both splints is identical. Proximal and distal pressure is applied volarly and the opposing middle force is applied dorsally.

IMMOBILIZATION SPLINTS

Simple thumb immobilization splints may involve one or more joints and may be fitted dorsally, volarly, or circumferentially (Fig. 10-1). Care should be taken to maintain correct ligamentous stress at each joint traversed, as well as full motion of the unsplinted joints. Straps placed at the level of the axis of joint rotation provide maximum mechanical purchase. Because many thumb immobilization splints have narrow configurations, contouring the material to half the segmental thickness provides splint strength. Circumferential thumb splints eliminate the need for counterforce straps at joints by providing opposing forces along the entire length of the segment (Fig. 10-2).

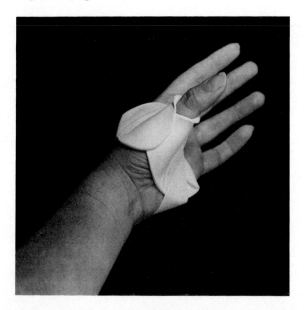

Fig. 10-2. Three-point pressure forces are disbursed along the length of the splinted segment in this circumferential metacarpal immobilization splint.

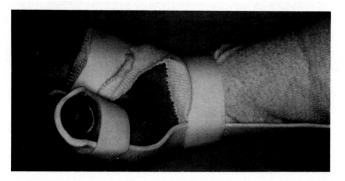

Fig. 10-3. This complex immobilization splint limits carpometacarpal, metacarpophalangeal, and interphalangeal joint thumb motion in addition to adjunctively immobilizing the wrist.

To control extrinsic thumb musculotendinous units, complex thumb immobilization splints statically position the wrist as an adjunctive measure to thumb immobilization. Wrist position may be used to increase or decrease the amount of tension on these units through alteration of the tenodesis effect. For optimum mechanical design the forearm trough should be at least two thirds the length of the forearm, and the C bar or thumb post should be of sufficient length to fully immobilize the intended segment while allowing unimpeded motion at the more distal unsplinted joints (Fig. 10-3).

MOBILIZATION SPLINTS

Severe hand injuries, particularly if a component of crush is involved, will often produce an insidious contracture of the first web space, which, if permitted to persist, will rapidly develop into a rigid adduction deformity markedly limiting thumb function.

Carpometacarpal level

Pathologic conditions at the carpometacarpal level will often result in a limited arc of motion of the first metacarpal with concomitant narrowing of the first web space. Any splint designed to maintain or increase the passive range of carpometacarpal motion must have its site of force application on the first metacarpal. Practically speaking, however, this is difficult because of the intervening soft tissue of the first web space. Many ill-conceived splints fitted with the intent of increasing carpometacarpal motion actually apply most of the rotatory force to the proximal phalanx, resulting in stretching of the ulnar collateral ligament of the metacarpophalangeal joint, radial deviation of the proximal phalanx, pressure over the radiometacarpal condyle, and instability of the thumb. Care must be taken to ensure that as much of the distal aspect of the first metacarpal is included in the splint as possible and that the primary site of the rotational force is directed toward the metacarpal. To decrease the amount of pressure on the first metacarpal, the area of force application can be widened to include the proximal phalanx, but this addition must not jeopardize the stability of the metacarpophalangeal joint by exerting a stretching force on the ulnar collateral ligament; in most instances the splint need not be extended distally beyond the interphalangeal flexion crease, thus allowing full motion of the distal phalanx. The splint should also be fitted proximal to the distal palmar flexion crease, permitting full metacarpophalangeal flexion of the adjacent digits. A static web spacer (Fig. 10-4) is one of the many splints that can be used to maintain the width of the first web space and ensure the most useful plane of motion of the thumb carpometacarpal joint.

Since the carpometacarpal joint of the thumb is a triaxial saddle articulation and possesses multiple planes of motion, the splinted position of the first metacarpal should be alternated from full extension to full abduction to minimize the possibility of shortening of the five carpometacarpal articular ligaments as described by Haines (1944) and Napier (1955). This may be accomplished through

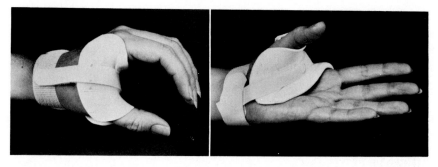

Fig. 10-4. A simple carpometacarpal mobilization splint such as this web spacer allows full range of motion of adjacent metacarpophalangeal joints while exerting rotational force to the distal aspect of the first metacarpal. Straps are designed to prevent distal migration of the splint. (From Fess, E.: Splinting for mobilization of the thumb. In Hunter, J. M., et al., editors: Rehabilitation of the hand, St. Louis, 1978, The C. V. Mosby Co.)

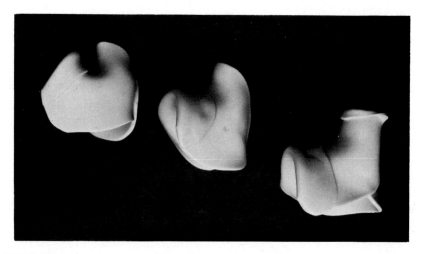

Fig. 10-5. Serial web spacers are widened every three or four days. (From Fess, E.: Splinting for mobilization of the thumb. In Hunter, J. M., et al., editors: Rehabilitation of the hand, St. Louis, 1978, The C. V. Mosby Co.)

the construction of two splints, one in full extension and the second in abduction, and through a carefully supervised exercise routine.

If a full passive range of motion is not present at the carpometacarpal joint, slow, progressive, inelastic traction may be applied through the use of serial web spacers (Fig. 10-5), which are changed and widened every three or four days. Progressive wedging of the thumb is continued until the passive measurements of abduction and extension duplicate those of the normal thumb or until the passive motion remains unchanged for three or four consecutive splint changes. In most instances, static serial web spacers are more effective than dynamic splinting for increasing the passive range of motion of the thumb carpometacarpal joint.

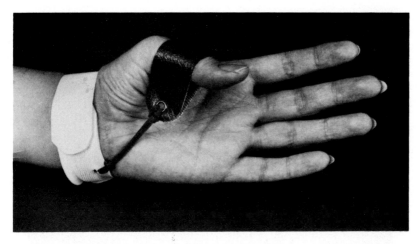

Fig. 10-6. The rigid low-temperature plastic component of the wristband is closely fitted around the ulnar border of the wrist to prevent the entire band from rotating as elastic traction is applied to the metacarpophalangeal joint. (From Fess, E.: Splinting for mobilization of the thumb. In Hunter, J. M., et al., editors: Rehabilitation of the hand, St. Louis, 1978, The C. V. Mosby Co.)

Metacarpophalangeal level

The middle joint in the important thumb chain is the metacarpophalangeal joint. At this level, stability is a more important consideration than mobility.

A wide discrepancy exists in the amount of thumb metacarpophalangeal motion found in the general population, with flexion ranging from only a few degrees to 90 degrees. It is apparent that the functional sequelae of limited or absent metacarpophalangeal motion is negligible if the joint is in extension and stable. The metacarpophalangeal joint of the thumb, unlike those of the fingers, tends to be more nearly of the ginglymoid or hinge type. In mobilizing this joint of the thumb, care should be taken to apply a rotational force perpendicular to the center of the axis of rotation of the metacarpophalangeal joint. If this concept is disregarded stretching of either the ulnar or radial collateral ligament may occur with resulting deviation of the proximal phalanx and metacarpophalangeal joint instability. The angle of the force should also be 90 degrees to the proximal phalanx.

A simple metacarpophalangeal flexion splint in the form of a wristband with flexion cuff (Fig. 10-6) is one of the least complicated means of facilitating thumb metacarpophalangeal flexion. It must be remembered that this splint affects motion at the thumb carpometacarpal joint, in addition to the metacarpophalangeal joint. Therefore, an incorrect force angle may cause medial or lateral rotation of the first metacarpal with stretching of the carpometacarpal ligaments and intra-articular pressure, as well as undue stressing of the metacarpophalangeal collateral ligaments and joint surfaces.

A compound metacarpophalangeal flexion splint allows the application of the full magnitude of the rotatory force on the metacarpophalangeal joint by stabilizing the thumb carpometacarpal joint (Fig. 10-7). Once again, attention must be directed toward ensuring that the force angle of approach is directed 90 degrees to the proximal phalanx and perpendicular to the center of the axis for rotation of the metacarpophalangeal joint.

Secondary wrist immobilization is a definitive characteristic of complex thumb mobilization splints. These splints may be fitted dorsally or volarly, and, as with the complex immobilization splints, wrist position through a tenodesis effect influences tension on the extrinsic thumb musculotendinous units. The dynamic assist or C bar should apply a 90-degree rotary force to the segment being mobilized; in the case of metacarpophalangeal or interphalangeal mobilization, the traction should also be perpendicular to the axis joint rotation (Fig. 10-8).

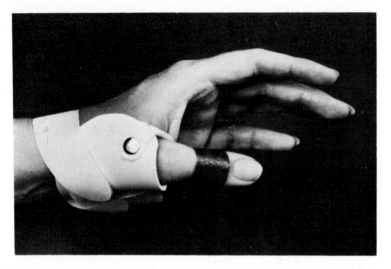

Fig. 10-7. Because of the immobilization of the carpometacarpal joint, the full effect of the traction is focused on the metacarpophalangeal joint in this compound splint. (From Fess, E.: Splinting for mobilization of the thumb. In Hunter, J. M., et al., editors: Rehabilitation of the hand, St. Louis, 1978, The C. V. Mosby Co.)

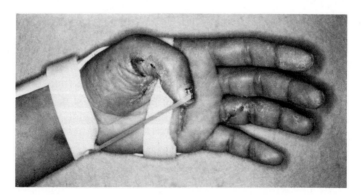

Fig. 10-8. This complex thumb flexion splint influences articular motion and extrinsic tendon excursion.

As with metacarpophalangeal joint mobilization in the companion digits, the most carefully designed and constructed splints may totally fail to overcome contracture (usually extension) despite the most vigorous efforts of both therapist and patient. It must be realized at the onset that in many instances this type of fixed deformity has such rigid underlying fibrosis and ligamentous pathologic conditions that no amount of splinting, however well conceived, can be expected to succeed. To avoid frustration by both parties, a realistic understanding of the possibility of failure is essential when the splinting program is initiated.

Interphalangeal level

Although strong interphalangeal joint motion is valuable to thumb performance, its absence is not critical, and almost all thumb functions are possible if there is a good carpometacarpal joint and perhaps some metacarpophalangeal joint motion. Since the interphalangeal joint of the thumb is a true uniaxial hinge articulation, the mechanical principles previously mentioned regarding mobilization of the thumb metacarpophalangeal joint are applicable to the mobilization of the thumb interphalangeal joint. For optimum results, the angle of approach should be 90 degrees to the distal phalanx of the thumb and perpendicular to the center of the axis of rotation of the interphalangeal joint.

A wristband and a fingernail clip (Fig. 10-9) mobilize the carpometacarpal, metacarpophalangeal, and interphalangeal joints of the thumb. In fitting this simple classification splint, care must be taken to check the angle of force application. The incorporation of all three joints of the thumb into the splint leaves little room for error and may tend to cause or accentuate deformity because of the multiple lever arms. The angle of approach of the rubber band must be perpendicular to the

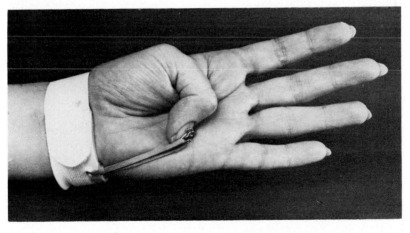

Fig. 10-9. A wristband with rigid ulnar component and fingernail clip enhances passive flexion of the carpometacarpal, metacarpophalangeal, and interphalangeal joints of the thumb. (From Fess, E.: Splinting for mobilization of the thumb. In Hunter, J. M., et al., editors: Rehabilitation of the hand, St. Louis, 1978, The C. V. Mosby Co.)

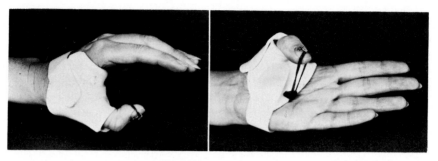

Fig. 10-10. This circumferential compound interphalangeal flexion splint allows the application of the elastic traction to affect only the distal thumb joint. The clip, a dressmaker's No. 2 hook, is attached with ethyl cyanoacrylate glue. (From Fess, E.: Splinting for mobilization of the thumb. In Hunter, J. M., et al., editors: Rehabilitation of the hand, St. Louis, 1978, The C. V. Mosby Co.)

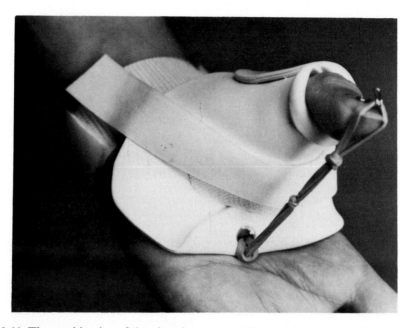

Fig. 10-11. The combination of thumb web spacer and fingernail clip allows for the simultaneous mobilization of carpometacarpal and interphalangeal joints. (From Fess, E.: Splinting for mobilization of the thumb. In Hunter, J. M., et al., editors: Rehabilitation of the hand, St. Louis, 1978, The C. V. Mosby Co.)

axis of rotation of the metacarpophalangeal and interphalangeal joints without causing transverse rotation of the first metacarpal.

A compound interphalangeal flexion splint (Fig. 10-10) may be employed to stabilize the carpometacarpal and metacarpophalangeal joints of the thumb, thus allowing for increased magnitude and accuracy of the application of the rotatory force at the interphalangeal joint, by way of a fingernail clip. To decrease the amount of pressure incurred by inhibiting motion at the carpometacarpal and metacarpophalangeal joints, this short opponens type of splint should be extended as far distally as possible along the proximal phalanx without interfering with full interphalangeal flexion. Room for complete flexion of the adjacent digital metacarpophalangeal joints and support of the transverse metacarpal arch should also be provided.

The fingernail clip should be attached to the center and proximal aspect of the thumbnail to eliminate the possibility of transverse rotation of the distal phalanx and to minimize the leverage effect of the nail on the proximal nail bed.

The techniques discussed in this chapter for splinting individual joints may be combined effectively for the simultaneous mobilization of multiple joints of the thumb. A web spacer, combined with a fingernail clip (Fig. 10-11), facilitates motion at both the carpometacarpal and interphalangeal joints. In designing and fitting this splint, it is necessary to be certain that the plastic fully extends around the proximal phalanx of the thumb, thus rendering the metacarpophalangeal joint immobile and diminishing the pressure on the volar aspect of the phalanx. Once again, the angle of approach of the rubber band should be at a 90-degree angle to the distal phalanx and perpendicular to the center of the axis of rotation of the interphalangeal joint. The metacarpophalangeal joints of the fingers should also be permitted a full range of motion into flexion.

SUMMARY

It is of utmost importance that thumb splints be created to provide functional position, stability, and at least basilar joint mobility. Although careful adherence to the basic design, mechanics, construction, and fit principles remains important, the thumb must be considered as a separate unique unit with splints used to carefully provide a maximum return of thumb participation in the important pinching and grasping activities of the hand. If done properly, the combination of splinting, exercise, and purposeful activity may help to minimize the disabling effect of disease and trauma to the thumb and enhance the results of surgery.

CHAPTER 11

Exercise and splinting for specific problems

This chapter is concerned with a number of frequently encountered clinical hand conditions and attempts to suggest the appropriate splinting approach to each problem. Although there may be considerable variation in the individual presentation of a particular hand problem, certain common features must be dealt with in each situation. Consideration of the underlying pathologic condition of each of these problems will be given, as well as an integrated program with emphasis on splinting provided to help restore the afflicted extremity to its best functional level. It should be clearly understood that, in most of these problems, isolated splinting will be much less effective than will a combination of splinting and exercise programs under the supervision of a knowledgeable physician-therapist team. It is therefore appropriate to include general exercise concepts in this chapter.

EXERCISE

To produce optimum results during hand rehabilitation, splinting and exercise must be carefully integrated. The application of an external device such as a hand splint may improve passive joint mobility but will do little to enhance the equally important active range of motion that must be provided by volutional use of strong forearm and hand muscles whose tendinous extensions have adhesion-free excursion and smooth gliding beds. Active motion through exercise and purposeful activity is the key to establishing and maintaining the functional capacity of a hand (Fig. 11-1).

The maximum passive range of motion of a joint must be realized before a corresponding range of active motion can be achieved. Splinting, therefore, is frequently employed as one of the initial treatment modalities when exercise alone is insufficient to attain an acceptable level of motion. A combination of appropriate hand splinting augmented with a structured and individualized exercise program may best provide for the restoration of the maximum functional potential in a given hand problem.

Since entire books are available that deal solely with the subject of exercise, the purpose of this chapter is not to compete with these works, but rather to re-

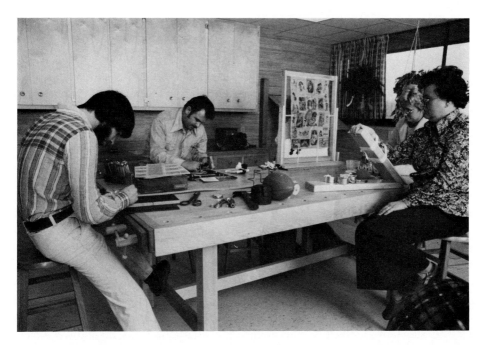

Fig. 11-1. Group interaction helps maintain enthusiasm and interest during the rehabilitative process. Patients are encouraged to use their afflicted hands in functional activities as soon as it is medically feasible.

view the fundamental concepts of exercise to produce a common framework of terminology and theory that may then be related to the clinical use of splinting of the upper extremity.

Basically, there are three types of exercise: (1) passive exercise, in which a joint is moved through an arc of motion by an external force without the assistance of active muscle contraction; (2) active exercise, in which joint movement is the result of physiologic muscle contraction; and (3) resistive exercise, in which an external opposing force is applied against the mobile segment of the joint as active motion is attempted. The focus of each type of exercise is centered on different anatomic structures, and the respective objectives and methods of implementation of each are significantly different.

Passive exercise

Passive exercise produces gliding of the articular surfaces and excursion of tendons and capsular structures through the use of externally applied forces such as manipulation techniques or traction devices. Hand splinting is an effective conservative means of attaining passive mobility and, when used appropriately, produces a gradual rearrangement or lengthening of the pericapsular structures and a disruption of adhesions through directed gentle traction. The small joints of the hand, with their delicate pericapsular ligamentous arrangement, are uniquely susceptible to stiffening and deformity resulting from direct trauma or chronic edema. Overzealous attempts to improve passive range of motion of a hand joint by overly tight elastic traction or poorly applied manual techniques may not only fail to improve motion, but may actually create further tissue damage and edema. Any passive method of joint mobilization should be carefully monitored with specific attention to patient discomfort, hand edema, and changes in the range of motion.

Active exercise

Active exercise through purposeful activity and individualized exercise routines produces joint motion effected by muscle contraction and resultant tendon excursion. Achievement of a functional level of active motion is dependent on the presence of adequate muscle strength and passively supple joints. Active range of motion may be considerably benefited by correctly implemented passive motion and splinting techniques that may mobilize arthrofibrosed joints and adherent tendons or lengthen myostatically shortened muscles or tight pericapsular structures. For joints whose diminished range of motion is secondary to an extrinsic tenodesis effect from tendon adhesion or muscle shortening rather than a pericapsular pathologic condition, the active improvement from passive mobilization efforts may be substantial. Because the application of traction has diminutive effects on motion at the musculotendinous level once the full passive mobility of a joint is established and the tenodesis effect minimized, splinting should not be relied on to further enhance active motion. Active exercise programs, however, may be aided by the splinting of adjacent (usually proximal) joints, particularly the wrist, to maximize tendon amplitude at a given joint or to use or negate the tenodesis effect. Repetitive attempts at active motion in the form of specific structured exercises and the use of the extremity in functional adapted and graded activities are the most productive means for increasing and maintaining strength and amplitude at the musculotendinous level (Fig. 11-2).

Resistive exercise

The purpose of resistive exercise is to produce sufficient muscle strength to allow maximum tendon excursion, full joint motion, and the execution of normal daily activities. This may be accomplished through purposeful graded activities and progressive resistive exercises. An external splinting force applied to a wrist or hand joint will have little appreciable effect on improving muscle strength, since it requires volutional effort programs to enhance power. In addition to strengthening muscles, resistive exercises may be used to provide a type of biofeedback to the patient, allowing increased awareness of the position and function of key muscle groups (Fig. 11-3). Resistive exercises may be used at many stages of rehabilitation but should not be relied on solely to increase the passive range of motion of stiffened joints. Mechanically, because of the angle of approach of a tendon to a given joint, the strength of a muscle is often lost in translational force when attempting active mobilization of a stiff joint (Fig. 11-4). From a physiologic view-

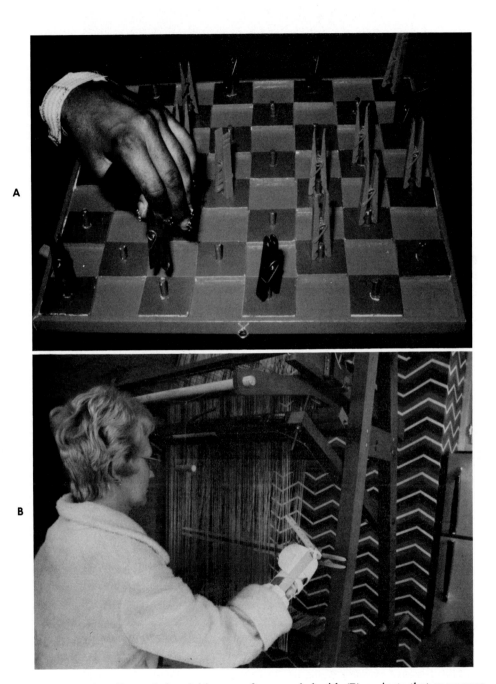

Fig. 11-2. A, Specific graded activities are often coupled with (**B**) projects that encourage gross motion of the entire extremity. (A courtesy Joan Farrell, O.T.R., Lauderhill, Florida.)

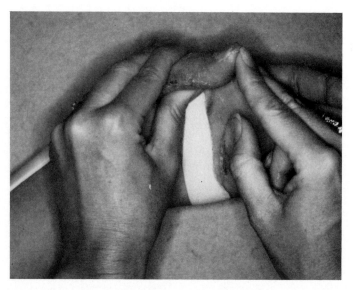

Fig. 11-3. Manual application of mild resistance to a segment as it is volutionally moved through its arc of motion may be used as a type of biofeedback.

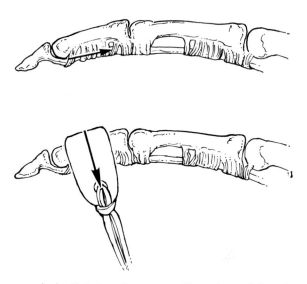

Fig. 11-4. Because extrinsic digital tendons normally run parallel to the phalanges, their force angle of approach to the joints they cross is not as mechanically advantageous as that which may be achieved by an externally positioned splint.

point, the musculotendinous unit cannot provide the long-term tension on the joint needed to cause pericapsular readjustment. Splinting will effect a more advantageous and sustained angle of pull because of its external position, producing better results with less force.

•   •   •

These three basic exercises may be effectively merged to meet the needs of the individual situation. For example, active assistive exercise is a combination of active and passive exercises in which the involved joint is moved actively as far as possible with passive completion of the remaining arc of motion.

A sequential program employing these basic types of exercise in a logical order will eliminate for the patient many hours of well-intentioned but nonproductive exercise. The achievement of passively supple joints is a prerequisite to the establishment of active range-of-motion and resistive exercises. It must be recognized that the active motion of a joint cannot be greater than its existing passive range of motion, and, regardless of the strength or amplitude of the involved musculotendinous unit, the absence of satisfactory passive joint motion will negate its functional effect. Adequate joint motion is dependent on a minimum of fair grade muscle strength. In the presence of resistance-producing tendon adhesions the involved musculature should be functioning on a good or normal level to effect excursion change.

Muscle atrophy, with or without myostatic contracture, will have a profound effect on the ultimate performance of a joint after it has been successfully mobilized. Therefore, it is extremely important to develop and maintain muscle strengthening exercises early in the rehabilitation process, often well in advance of the ability of the muscle to effect appreciable motion at the joints it crosses. It is no less important that these strengthening exercises be carried out in all extremity muscle groups and not limited to those whose weakness or atrophy is obvious.

AMPUTATION

Unfortunately, amputation of portions of a digit or hand frequently occurs after hand injury. From both a psychologic and functional standpoint it is important that all efforts be devoted to rapidly restoring the amputation victim to a productive status.

Splinting of a hand that has undergone amputation of a part is usually directed toward one of three purposes: (1) the maintenance of motion of uninvolved joints, (2) protective splinting to the area of amputation, and (3) functional splinting to improve prehension patterns. Emphasis is placed on prevention of adhesions and the return of maximum function commensurate with the particular loss. The unnecessary stiffening of unaffected digital joints after amputation usually reflects a failure to establish motion programs at an early stage. The patient with a digital amputation is often reluctant to remove bandages and resume hand motion because of self-consciousness and fear of pain.

Because amputation often results in generalized edema of the hand and the potential stiffness of the remaining adjacent joints is increased, splinting may be required to augment exercise programs. In the early postamputation phase, joints in adjacent digits readily respond to uncomplicated traction devices, such as wide rubber bands and glove rubber bands for flexion and three point fixation splints for extension. Joints proximal to the site of amputation may be more resilient to the establishment and maintenance of good passive and active range of motion, requiring more complicated splints to attain an acceptable level of motion.

To encourage early use of the hand in purposeful activity, a temporary protective splint may be designed to fit over a distal aspect of the remaining digit. This prevents unintentional bumping of the tender stump and allows more uninhibited use of the hand as healing progresses. These splints are frequently fitted over dressings and should be removed during inactive periods for cleaning and to allow ventilation. Care should be taken to prevent wound maceration from improper splint wear.

The potential for dependence on a protective splint should be acknowledged, and measures taken to gradually wean the patient from the splint as self-confidence increases and area sensitivity decreases. The initiation of a desensitization program is often instrumental in hastening unprotected hand use (Fig. 11-5). Persistent hypersensitivity at the healed site of amputation may be indicative of unresolved problems such as retained terminal neuromas; evaluation by a physician should be requested.

Functional splinting of a partially amputated hand permits accomplishment of

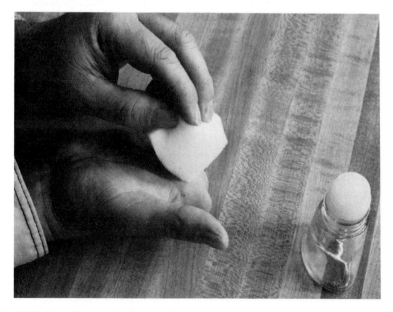

Fig. 11-5. Initiation of an early desensitization program often facilitates functional use of the hand after amputation.

special occupational tasks (Fig. 11-6). Splint designs range from relatively simple to extremely complicated, depending on specific anatomic loss and patient requirements. Durability of the splint is often a key factor and may necessitate collaboration with an orthotist (Fig. 11-7).

It is important that an excellent rapport is established with the hand amputation patient. The loss of a body part is a severe psychologic blow, regardless of the level, and the patient must be gently brought to understand the importance of accepting the loss and devoting efforts to the maintenance and restoration of maximum function in the remaining hand.

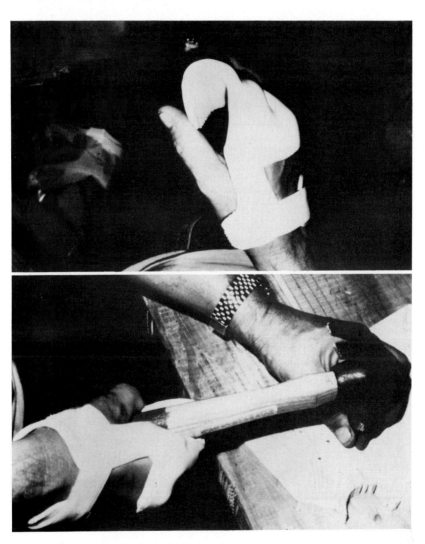

Fig. 11-6. Provision of an adapted gripping surface against which the thumb could oppose allowed this patient to grasp and use a hammer. (Courtesy Joan Farrell, O.T.R., Lauderhill, Florida.)

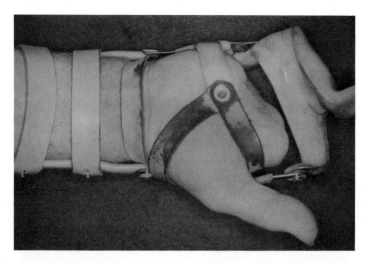

Fig. 11-7. Because this man required splint durability that could not be attained with routine splinting materials, he was referred to an orthotist who specializes in metal hand braces.

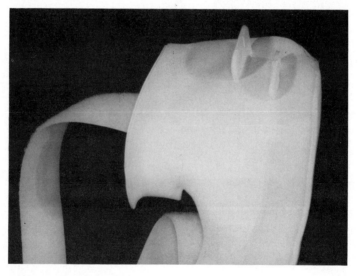

Fig. 11-8. Deviation bars in the finger pan of this night splint maintain the fingers of a rheumatoid arthritic patient in correct alignment.

ARTHRITIS

Controversy surrounds the subject of splinting of the rheumatoid hand. Some physicians believe strongly that the application of hand splints plays a major role in preventing or retarding the insidious deforming process of the disease by maintaining correct joint alignment and decreasing stress on the pericapsular structures (Fig. 11-8). Others state that, although splints cannot inhibit the disease process and its relentless sequelae, their use may enhance hand function (Fig. 11-9); still others maintain that splinting the rheumatoid hand is of little value.

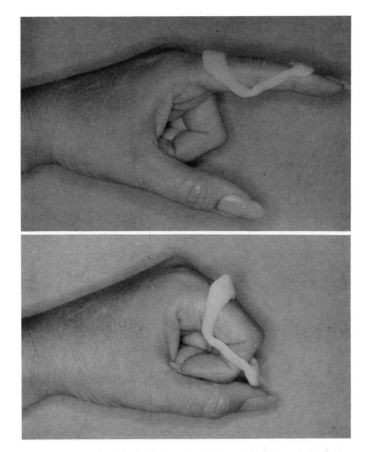

Fig. 11-9. This simple proximal interphalangeal joint extension block splint designed by Irene Hollis, O.T.R., Chapel Hill, North Carolina, prevents hyperextension and lateral instability of the proximal interphalangeal joint without interfering with digital flexion.

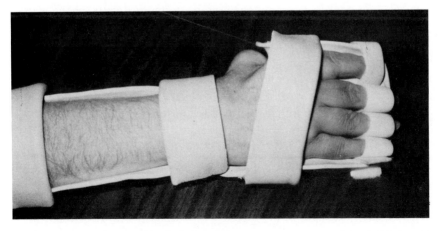

Fig. 11-10. Immobilization of acutely inflamed joints in the rheumatoid arthritic hand helps alleviate pain. (Courtesy Joan Farrell, O.T.R., Lauderhill, Florida.)

Despite this lack of agreement, few dispute the fact that temporary immobilization of affected joints during acute inflammatory stages helps alleviate pain and permits continued use of uninvolved joints (Fig. 11-10). Severely impaired joints that contribute more stability than mobility to overall hand dexterity may also be immobilized in positions of function.

Because of the slowly progressive development of rheumatoid hand deformities, functional adaptation by the patient to the gradual structural collapse occurs almost without recognition. Splinting directed toward enhancing hand function should be thoroughly and objectively evaluated. Although a splint may improve joint alignment, the resulting immediate positional change often causes further limitation of coordination and dexterity, requiring the patient to adapt to the splint in addition to the deformity. Unless quantitative improvement occurs in hand use, one should suppress the impulse to load these patients with splints and gadgets that, despite their expense and clever design, will ultimately be discarded. Furthermore, one should remember that long immobilization of joints will often result in a disuse weakening of the muscle that move the joints, compounding the strength loss already present in the arthritic patient. In the last analysis, the decision regarding the use of splints on the wrist and hand of an arthritic patient must be based on direct input from the patient with regard to pain relief, functional improvement, and perhaps the slowing of deformity progression.

The disabling hand involvement in the arthritic patient is usually bilateral. When splints are fitted, special adaptations are often required to permit independent application and removal. Loops or tabs on straps facilitate prehension in patients whose grasp is weak, and adjustable straps on the nondominant side splint are often required to provide independent use of bilateral immobilization splints such as resting pans or night splints. The use of distal loops or finger deviation bars on the finger pan of a resting splint provides individual digital control that often allows the patient to slip the fingers into and out of the splint without additional adjustment. When a splint fits circumferentially, as with some metacarpophalangeal ulnar deviation, swan-neck, and boutonniere splints, changes in external joint circumference should be anticipated, and appropriate splint adaptations made. If this is not done, the splint may be difficult to remove after several hours of wear. Close observation of the splinted extremity is particularly important in arthritis where friable skin and subcutaneous atrophy result in an increased vulnerability to pressure. Patients should be taught to remove the splints frequently and to inspect their skin for any signs of irritation.

ARTHROPLASTY

Joints destroyed by trauma or disease may undergo arthroplasty procedures in an attempt to restore pain-free function. Techniques vary considerably and many modifications have been made over the years to try and produce consistently satisfactory results. Excision of destroyed joint surfaces, with or without the interposition of autogenous soft tissues or inert biocompatible materials such as silicone, rubber polyethylene, or stainless steel comprise the basic surgical techniques employed in these restoration procedures. Concomitant soft tissue reconstruction is often the most important part of these procedures, and the postoperative exercise and splinting regimen must be worked out with careful consideration of the exact surgical methods used.

After arthroplasty, it is necessary to protect ligament and tendon reconstruction while allowing controlled motion in the flexion-extension plane. By permitting motion in the anteroposterior plane and preventing it in the lateral or coronal plane, one can model the developing pseudocapsular fibrins around an arthroplasty to impart both mobility and stability in the desired directions. The process must be carefully monitored because of the great individual variation in scar formation and collagen maturation. Frequent changes in exercise programs and splinting techniques may be necessary to respond to the performance of a given arthroplasty. Certainly no standard postoperative regimen will be applicable for all patients.

The type of splint applied and the ensuing exercise program are dependent on the specific joint replaced and on the type of prosthesis used. Some prostheses permit sagittal plane motion only, whereas the inherent flexibility of other designs allows motion in several planes. The more flexible implants rely heavily on surgical repair of periarticular structures and the programmed development of a pseudocapsule to control the direction of joint motion and to prevent recurrent deformity.

Metacarpophalangeal joint

Metacarpophalangeal prostheses differ considerably in design. Silicone implants, which lack inherent stability, require splints that provide radially directed metacarpophalangeal traction to prevent recurrent ulnar drift in addition to dynamic flexion and extension forces (Fig. 11-11). The accompnaying exercise program emphasizes early active motion in extension slings and flexion splinting initiated at approximately the third week after surgery (Fig. 11-12). Splinting for correction of the pronation or medial rotation deformity of the index and long fingers may be implemented through the addition of a two-sling force couple, a supinatory splint, or a Velcro supination attachment device (Fig. 11-13). Numerous variations on these exercise and splinting programs exist throughout the country, but most adhere to radial deviation with alternating flexion-extension and introduce active motion in the splint within the first week after surgery.

Rigid articulated metacarpophalangeal prostheses that permit sagittal motion necessitate splints which augment flexion and extension but do not require the element of radial deviation traction.

Simple interphalangeal immobilization splints may also be beneficial after metacarpophalangeal arthroplasty. These splints restrict distal finger joint motion and allow the full active extrinsic tendon excursion to be directed to the metacarpophalangeal joints (Fig. 11-14). This concept is helpful when confronted with a patient whose proximal interphalangeal joints are essentially normal and whose

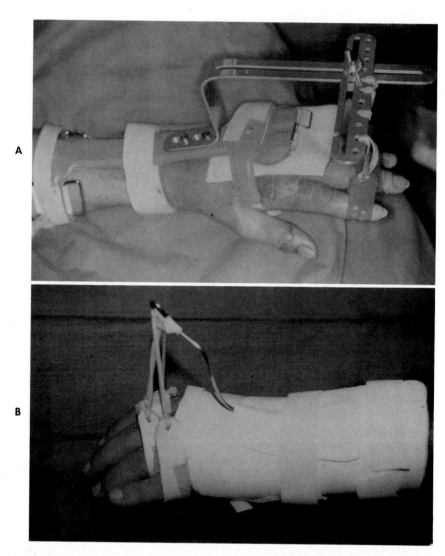

Fig. 11-11. Controlled radial extension may be accomplished through (**A**) an adjustable outrigger or (**B**) progressively longer rubber bands attached to a stationary radially placed extension outrigger. (**B** courtesy Cynthia Philips, O.T.R., Boston, Massachusetts.)

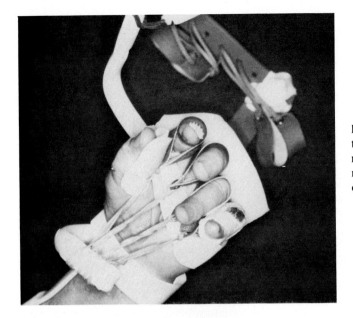

Fig. 11-12. Depending on the extent of the surgical repair, the flexion assists may also be directed radially.

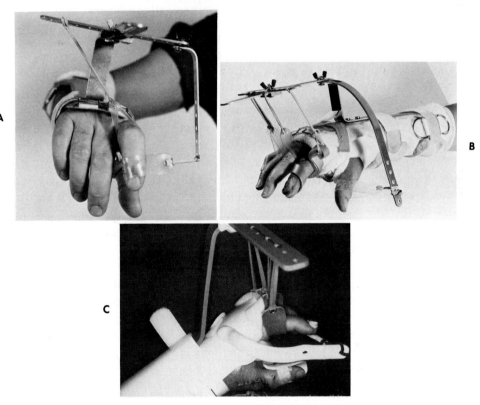

Fig. 11-13. The use of (**A**) a two-sling force couple, (**B**) a supinatory splint, or (**C**) a supination outrigger with a Velcro fingernail attachment device helps prevent the recurrence of a pronation deformity of the index or long finger. (**A** and **B** from Swanson, A. B., Swanson, G. de G., and Leonard, J.: Postoperative rehabilitation program in flexible implant arthroplasty of the digits. In Hunter, J. M., et al., editors: Rehabilitation of the hand, St. Louis, 1978, The C. V. Mosby Co.)

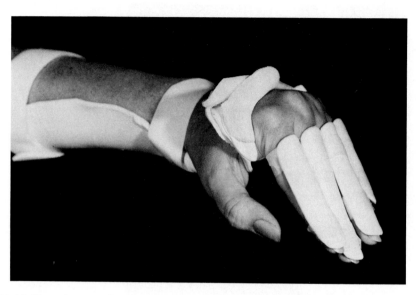

Fig. 11-14. Dorsal "gutter" splints immobilize the interphalangeal joints and focus motion produced by extrinsic tendon excursion on the metacarpophalangeal joints.

efforts at active postoperative metacarpophalangeal motion are frustrated by a tendency to waste the long tendon amplitude at the uninvolved joints.

Proximal interphalangeal joint

The splinting involved in a proximal interphalangeal replacement arthroplasty procedure is less complicated than that employed at the metacarpophalangeal level. It usually requires simple or compound flexion and extension splints, rather than a complex type, which immobilizes the wrist as an adjunctive measure. Because the proximal interphalangeal joint is normally limited to sagittal plane motion, care must be taken when applying traction to maintain a pull that is perpendicular to the center of the axis of rotation. If this is not accomplished, unequal stress on the collateral ligaments may occur with resulting ulnar or radial deviation of the middle phalanx. Timing of the initiation of active motion is dependent on the presence of associated tendon or ligamentous repairs. Flexion deformities often require surgical repair of the extensor mechanism, necessitating joint immobilization for approximately three weeks before active and passive motion may be initiated. The need for immobilization after a resection arthroplasty procedure with a preexisting proximal interphalangeal extension deformity is usually not present, allowing early mobilization of the implant. Alternating flexion and extension splinting may be interspersed with frequent active exercise periods to achieve optimum joint function.

Wrist

An articulated wrist mobilization splint may be employed to increase the sagittal motion during the postoperative phase of a wrist replacement arthroplasty

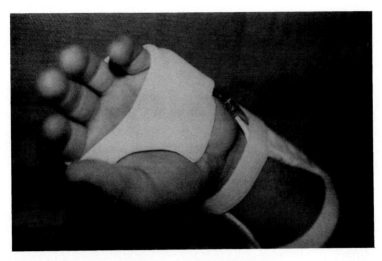

Fig. 11-15. The splint and anatomic axes of rotation must be accurately aligned with each other when fitting this postoperative articulated wrist splint. (Courtesy Cynthia Philips, O.T.R., Boston, Massachusetts.)

procedure (Fig. 11-15). If this simple category splint is used, it is of importance to align the splint axis with the anatomic axis of rotation. A 90-degree angle of pull to the metacarpals, which is also perpendicular to the center of the axis of rotation, is important to obtain maximal use of the magnitude of the traction and to apply equal amounts of force to the ulnar and radial structures of the wrist. Active and passive exercises and graded purposeful activity should be used in conjunction with wrist arthroplasty mobilization splinting.

CAPSULOTOMY/CAPSULECTOMY

Capsulectomy involves the surgical division (capsulotomy) or excision (capsulectomy) of a portion of the collateral ligaments of a digital joint with normal articular surfaces but limited passive motion because of contracted periarticular ligamentous structures. Although a substantial improvement of motion may be reliably anticipated at the metacarpophalangeal level, the results of a capsulectomy procedure at the proximal interphalangeal joint are less predictable. Mobilization efforts are usually initiated within one to seven days postoperatively. These efforts should involve aggressive splinting techniques on the part of the therapist and exercise programs for the patient.

Preoperative splinting and exercises are designed to attain as much passive joint motion as possible, enhancing the postoperative arc of motion and assuring adhesion-free tendon excursion essential to the active maintenance of passively improved postoperative motion. Splints should be adapted to meet individual patient variations, and the decision as to the type of splint to be applied depends on the presence or absence of wrist-produced tenodesis effect. If the limitation is

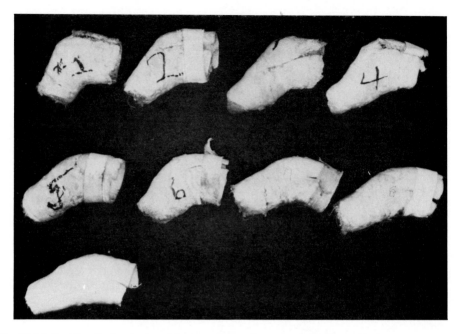

Fig. 11-16. Serial cylinder casts, which are changed every two or three days, may be used to enhance passive interphalangeal joint motion before a capsulotomy/capsulectomy procedure is undertaken. Cylinder casts are also effective in maintaining postoperative motion once the initial edema subsides and the incision is healed.

purely articular, simple or compound splints will suffice (Fig. 11-16). Complex splints with adjunctive wrist immobilization are required to control the effects of wrist position on distal joints in the presence of extrinsic tendon adhesions or poor postural habits that unfavorably affect digital joint mechanics.

Splinting of a joint that has undergone a capsulectomy procedure is utilized to maintain the motion gained from the combined preoperative and operative efforts. Because of the potential recurrence of extension contractures, the metacarpophalangeal joints are usually splinted with devices that encourage joint flexion. Extension is often more difficult to regain than is flexion in the capsulectomized proximal interphalangeal joint. For this reason extension splinting, which is interspersed with frequent exercise periods and limited flexion splinting, may need to be prolonged to prevent recurrence of deformity. It is important that postcapsulectomy splinting and exercise programs be frequently reevaluated by members of the hand rehabilitation team during the first two or three postoperative months, and appropriate changes be instigated to ensure optimum results. One should emphasize to the patient undergoing these difficult joint mobilization procedures that the tendency for restiffening of the involved joints is great and that splinting may be necessary for many months.

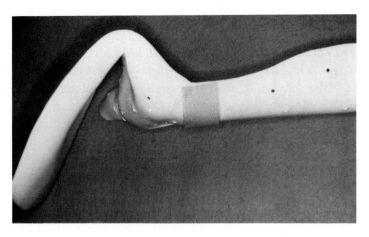

Fig. 11-17. Safe position splints are frequently used during the early stages of burn, crush, or frostbite injuries.

CRUSH, BURN, AND COLD INJURIES

Although emanating from dissimilar causes, extensive soft tissue damage resulting in crush, burn, and frostbite injuries often requires similar conservative treatment. Hand splinting requirements after these injuries depend on the site and extent of tissue damage. When a major portion of the hand is involved, early use of a safe position splint alternated with exercise will facilitate preservation of collateral ligament length by maintaining joint postures that place these ligaments at near-maximum tension (Fig. 11-17).

Philosophies regarding optimum thumb position in a safe position splint differ. Full thumb abduction is advocated by some, whereas full extension is preferred by others. The key concept involved, however, is to maintain maximum passive range of motion at the first carpometacarpal joint and to adapt the splint to meet the individual requirements of the patient. To prevent the occurrence of additional arthrofibrotic changes in a hand already predisposed to swelling and stiffness, the use of this complex finger immobilization splint must be accompanied by frequent periods of passive and active exercises to the wrist and digital joints. As the extent of the injury becomes more apparent and additional splinting is required to maintain passive motion of specific joints, the use of a safe position splint may be alternated with mobilization splints or may be used only at night in deference to daytime exercise and mobility splinting.

Splints fitted on hands with soft tissue loss or damage must be altered at the design stage to adapt for the presence of surface defects, skin grafts, and draining areas. Underlying fractures are often present in this type of injury, and protruding internal fixation wires may also represent problems prejudicial to the achievement of a congruous splint fit. To enhance cleanliness and decrease the chance of tissue maceration from the presence of excessive moisture, splints may be fitted over several layers of light bandage. To ensure consistent and contiguous splint application, care must be taken to keep these dressings to a minimum. Padding is usually considered inappropriate in splints used on hands that have sustained extensive soft tissue damage because it tends to become contaminated with tissue exudate. The use of wide straps diminishes the possibility of circumferential constriction with the resultant propagation of increased edema.

FRACTURES

Trauma resulting in fracture of the small bones of the hand is one of the most commonly encountered injuries of the upper extremity. Fractures of the distal phalanx occur most frequently, followed by metacarpal, proximal phalangeal, and finally middle phalangeal fractures. The potential functional loss from this type of injury may be underestimated. Even if fracture healing occurs uneventfully, residual joint stiffness may become a serious factor in limiting composite hand function.

It has been shown by Strickland et al. (1979) that fracture immobilization beyond four weeks has a dramatically unfavorable effect on digital performance, although no clear-cut evidence is available to indicate that mobilization before the third week has any profound effect on the final range of motion. A patient age of over 50, fracture comminution, and, perhaps most importantly, associated tendon injuries also have a strongly detrimental effect on the ultimate digital function after fracture.

In the presence of a fracture, it is important to maintain the mobility of adjacent joints and digits to prevent magnification of the original injury through the development of secondary periarticular pathology. Internal fixation of the fracture with Kirschner wires or pins often eliminates the need to immobilize uninvolved joints and allows early mobilization of the hand, which is the key to preventing residual joint stiffness.

Splints should be designated to forestall the insidious development of deformity caused by edema and accompanying arthrofibrosis. Because the mechanical and physiologic repercussions of a fracture differ according to the severity of the injury, site of the fracture, quality of reduction, and method of immobilization used, each patient must be objectively evaluated and splint and exercise program created to meet the specific needs. The splint(s) should also be adapted to support the fractured segment and avoid protruding fixation pins. Complex splints with adjunctive wrist immobilization usually are not required in treating stable phalangeal fractures but may be of use with metacarpal fractures or unstable finger fractures where wrist control can lessen deforming tendon forces. It is not uncommon to splint for both flexion and extension of adjacent joints of a segment that has sustained a fracture.

Tendon injuries associated with phalangeal fractures have a particularly prejudicial effect because of the tendency for the tendon to become strongly adherent to the site of fracture healing. This obligatory loss of tendon amplitude, most often involving the extensor mechanism or flexor superficialis over the proximal phalanx or profundus over the middle phalanx, will severely limit distal joint excursion by virtue of its check-rein effect. In these instances it is extremely dangerous to rely on strong manipulative or dynamic traction techniques to improve digital joint motion because the restrictive adhesions may be so strong that tendon rupture or attenuation may occur, resulting in irreparable consequences. More gentle range-of-motion techniques are indicated here with consideration for early surgical lysis with or without capsulectomy when a strong tendon-bone bond is apparent.

The presence of associated ligament or neurovascular injury considerably alters the mode of conservative treatment. Consultation among members of the hand rehabilitation team is of paramount importance to establish goals and guidelines for postreduction management.

PEDIATRICS

In addition to the basic principles of design, mechanics, construction, and fit, variables exist that should be taken into consideration when working with pediatric patients. These variables may be incorporated and adapted according to the specific age and capabilities of the child being treated.

Because of the seemingly limitless physical activity of growing children, their splints must be solidly constructed of highly durable materials that are nontoxic and easily cleaned (Fig. 11-18). They should also be designed to remain in place on the extremity, and in case of an infant or young child, the splint should be difficult to remove except by an adult.

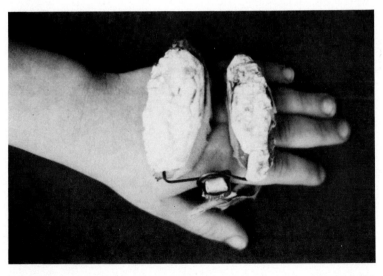

Fig. 11-18. Splinting materials used in children's splints should be durable and nontoxic. The plastic portion of this Orthoplast and spring-wire splint is almost unrecognizable because of the patient's habit of chewing on it.

Parents must be instructed as to proper splint care and wearing procedures. It may also be helpful to share this information with teachers and others who are frequently responsible for the child's care. Experience has shown that a combination of verbal and written guidelines produces less confusion than do verbal instructions alone.

During the fitting phase of splint fabrication, the child's anxiety may be diminished by allowing him to play with material scraps or by making up games or stories to promote cooperation. Drawing a face or design on the completed splint is also a successful enticement to encourage the child's acceptance of the splint (Fig. 11-19).

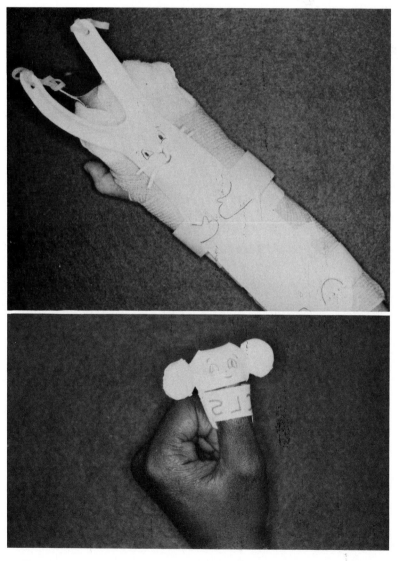

Fig. 11-19. Imagination and humor can entice a child to cooperate in the splinting program.

Although these "extras" may be initially time consuming, they ultimately result in the production of a more effective splint and improved results because of a cooperative patient and well-informed family.

PERIPHERAL NERVE INJURIES

The potential for the restoration of optimum hand function after peripheral nerve injuries of the upper extremity depends on the preservation of good passive joint motion. It is also necessary to protect periarticular structures and denervated musculature by avoiding improper positioning of the partially paralyzed extremity. In the presence of existing deformity, splints may be designed to restore passive mobility to digital joints. Adapted to the individual requirements of the patient, these splints may range from uncomplicated wide rubber bands to complex multifunction splints. Once free gliding of articular surfaces has been established, maintenance and positioning splints may be used until reinnervation occurs or until tendon transfer procedures are carried out to restore balance to the hand. These positioning splints should be used in conjunction with a good exercise program and serve to prevent deformity resulting from the unopposed antagonists of the paralyzed muscles as well as to position the hand for use while awaiting nerve regeneration. The splints may assume predictable configurations based on the nerve(s) involved and must be light and easily applied without excessive components, or they will not be worn.

In the supple hand, the need for protective splinting varies according to the type of lesion and the inherent laxity of the ligamentous structure of the individual hand. Not all patients who have sustained ulnar nerve injuries proceed to develop the classic claw hand posture of hyperextension of the fourth and fifth metacarpophalangeal joints and concomitant interphalangeal flexion. Some have unusually firm volar plate restraint at the metacarpophalangeal joints and are not predisposed to hyperextension deformities, despite the lack of intrinsic opposition to the long extensor muscles. All patients with total loss of radial nerve innervation to the wrist and digital extensors will develop a wrist drop and require external support to properly position the hand, both to avoid deformity and allow function.

Splinting requirements for each type of nerve loss are fairly predictable and will be considered.

Median nerve

The median nerve provides the critical sensory perception to the volar surface of the hand with the exception of the small finger and half of the ring. This nerve is also responsible for innervation of the pronator muscles, the radial wrist flexor, the superficial flexors of all digits, profundus flexion of the index and long fingers, and the long flexor of the thumb. At a more distal level the median nerve innervates the thenar muscles whose function is abduction and opposition. High median nerve lesions, therefore, are more disabling than is interruption at the wrist level, with the former affecting extrinsic as well as intrinsic digital function.

Splinting of median nerve injuries is dependent on the level of lesion. Emphasis is placed on maintenance of passive mobility of the involved joints and enhancement of function. High interruption may require splints that assist finger flexion as well as opposition of the thumb. Emphasis may be reduced to the prevention of thumb web contractures after more distal loss. An understanding of each patient's functional capacity and substitution patterns is important before a splint design is initiated. For example, many patients whose long thumb flexor or short abductor and opponens action has been lost will achieve adequate thumb use through substitution of the abductor pollicis longus, flexor pollicis brevis (deep head), and adductor pollicis.

Radial nerve

A high-level radial nerve injury results in loss of active wrist, thumb, and finger extension and a weakening of supination and thumb abduction. Because the wrist provides the key to hand function at the digital level, the loss of the ability to properly position the hand in extension markedly weakens grasp and diminishes coordination. The coexisting deficit of metacarpophalangeal extension presents a less significant problem because the intrinsic muscles provide active extension of the interphalangeal joints.

The most important objective in splinting a high radial nerve injury is to support the wrist in extension, enhancing hand function and preventing overstretching of the extensor muscle groups. For most patients the use of a simple wrist cock-up splint is sufficient to allow satisfactory hand use. Complex splints with extension outrigger attachments are, for the most part, excessive and should be used only in situations in which full digital extension is required for successful accomplishment of given tasks.

Ulnar nerve

The ulnar nerve, with its important intrinsic innervation, is largely responsible for delicate coordinated movements of the hand. In addition, it also influences

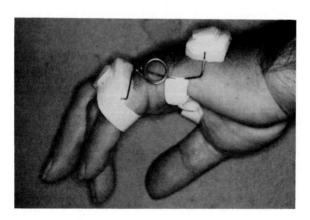

Fig. 11-20. This ulnar nerve paralysis splint prevents hyperextension at the metacarpophalangeal joints of the ring and small fingers.

flexion of the ring and small fingers and ulnar deviation and flexion of the wrist. Disruption of the ulnar nerve may result in the development of a claw deformity with metacarpophalangeal joint hyperextension and interphalangeal joint flexion of the fourth and fifth digits. Loss of small finger abduction and opposition and adduction of the thumb with the resultant weakness of pinch also accompanies ulnar paralysis.

The goals of splinting a hand that has sustained an ulnar nerve lesion are directed toward the attainment and maintenance of full passive motion and the improvement of hand function. Existing joint limitations, often at the proximal interphalangeal joint of the ring or small finger, must be corrected before maintenance or functional splinting programs may be initiated. Splints designed to correct deformity should be specifically created to meet individual needs and should be changed to maintain optimum mechanical purchase as joint motion improves. When full passive motion has been established, or if the hand is supple at the time of initial examination, preventive splinting may commence.

Positioning the fourth and fifth metacarpophalangeal joints in slight flexion allows the amplitude of the extrinsic digital extensor muscles to act effectively on the interphalangeal joints. Numerous splint designs accomplish this objective, but one of the most acceptable is a three-point dynamic piano wire splint described by Wynn Parry (1973). Adaptation of this splint to the use of low-temperature materials for the dorsal and palmar metacarpal bars and dorsal phalangeal bar makes construction and fitting easier (Fig. 11-20). Preventive splints may be used until nerve regeneration is complete, or until tendon transfer procedures are done.

Combined nerve injuries

Damage to multiple nerves of the upper extremity is not uncommon, and the resulting potential for the development of deformity is, of course, magnified.

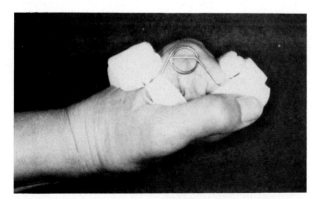

Fig. 11-21. This spring-wire splint prevents metacarpophalangeal hyperextension of the second through fifth metacarpophalangeal joints without interfering with digital flexion. It is one of several splints that may be used with combined ulnar and median nerve lesions.

Splinting programs should continue to incorporate the concepts previously mentioned for each individual injury, with even more care taken to monitor progress and make necessary adaptations as changes occur (Fig. 11-21).

The splinting of peripheral nerve injuries should be augmented with individually designed exercise programs that promote the maintenance of active and passive motion and enhance hand dexterity. Although the goals of these two programs will be almost identical, each brings a unique contribution to minimizing the resultant disability and in conjunction with one another provide an integrated and practical approach to hand rehabilitation. Each splint and exercise routine should also be interspersed with periodic objective reevaluation sessions to provide appropriate guidelines for alteration of programs, which allow for continued functional progress.

QUADRIPLEGIA

Splinting of the quadriplegic hand is dependent on the level of the spinal cord lesion. Extremities that lack innervation above the seventh cervical nerve (C7) level often require the development of a passive or active tenodesis function for grasp, whereas those at C7 have active gross grasp and release through innervated extrinsic flexors and extensors. The intrinsic muscles of the hand are usually innervated at the first thoracic nerve level, allowing normal hand function.

Fifth cervical nerve. Patients with lesions at this level usually have active elbow flexion and deltoid shoulder movements, allowing gross positioning of the forearm and hand. Paralyzed wrist and hand musculature necessitates external wrist support in the form of a simple wrist immobilization splint to provide distal stability of the extremity. Accommodation of the splint to serve as the basis of attachment for adapted equipment is important to establishing independence in activities of daily living. Thumb carpometacarpal position and passive motion may be maintained through web spacers that alternately position the thumb in abduction and extension. Wrist and thumb splints are often combined (Fig. 11-22).

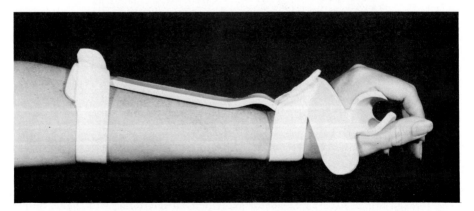

Fig. 11-22. A long opponens splint with a C bar is one of several designs that may be used to stabilize the wrist and maintain the first web space of a C5 spinal cord lesion patient.

If the patient is a candidate for an externally powered splint, the development of a passive tenodesis hand may be considered (next section). Most externally powered splints create a gross grasp or pinch by providing a power source to drive a conventional wrist-operated tenodesis splint. Power sources vary, as do triggering mechanisms (Fig. 11-23).

Sixth cervical nerve. In spinal cord lesions at this level, shoulder and elbow motions are stronger, resulting in more coordinated extremity positioning, but active elbow extension is absent. The important wrist extensors are spared, permitting a tenodesis hand in which grasp is achieved through an active wrist extension–passive finger flexion pattern. Tenodesis hands may be maximally developed through carefully supervised exercise and splinting programs. Exercises are oriented toward allowing controlled extrinsic flexor tightness to occur while maintaining passive range of motion of the wrist and digits. Finger extension exercises are performed with the wrist in flexion, and finger flexion exercises are carried out with the wrist in extension. Splints designed to augment these patterns are used to rein-

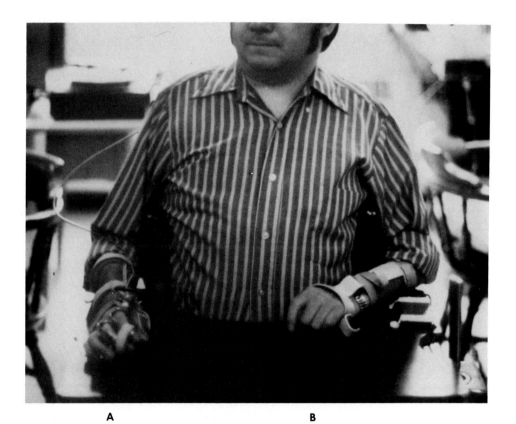

A   B

Fig. 11-23. A, A battery-powered external orthosis allows this C5 quadriplegic patient to grasp and release objects. **B,** The orthosis is triggered when the patient touches his watchband to the copper plate mounted on his lap board. (United States patent No. 3967321: Ryan, Fess, Babcock, et al.)

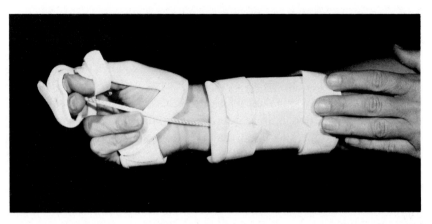

Fig. 11-24. This tenodesis splint produces passive approximation of the index and long fingers to the thumb through active wrist extension.

force the tenodesis motion in functional activities (Fig. 11-24). As habit patterns become established, gradual weaning from the splint may be encouraged, allowing increasingly independent tenodesis hand use.

Moberg (1975) describes a method for using the wrist extensors to enhance flexor hinge key grip of the thumb. Splinting for this procedure involves maintenance of passive mobility of the thumb carpometacarpal and metacarpophalangeal joints preoperatively and protective splinting of the transfer during the early postoperative mobilization phase. A small web spacer may occasionally be required to maintain carpometacarpal motion as postoperative time increases.

Seventh cervical nerve. Patients with lesions at this level usually have gross active finger flexion and extension but lack the intrinsic musculature that allows fine hand coordination and dexterity. Splinting and exercise programs are directed toward maintenance of passive joint range of motion with emphasis on thumb carpometacarpal mobility and prevention of extension deformities at the metacarpophalangeal joints. Splinting to position the thumb in opposition may be used to enhance prehension of small objects.

REPLANTATION

The splinting program employed with patients who have undergone replantation procedures emphasizes the attainment and maintenance of motion in adjacent uninvolved digits and in the replanted segment. Because of the obligatory immobilization of repaired structures to promote healing, the interval between the initiation of each type of splinting is often several weeks.

Depending on the level of severance, viability status of the replant, and size of the postoperative dressing, splinting and exercises may be carried out on joints not included in the dressing within the first postoperative week, providing the mobilization does not stress repaired structures.

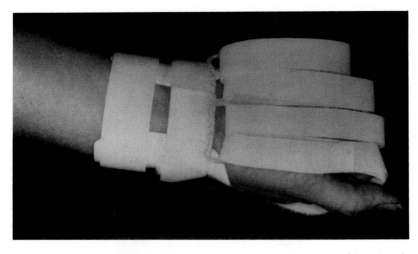

Fig. 11-25. The wristband of this simple finger flexion splint has been widened to decrease pressure from the splint on the distal forearm.

Splinting of the replanted segment may begin as early as three weeks after replantation. With gutter splints providing external support to internally fixated fractures, gentle mobilization traction designed according to individual requirements may be initiated. Because of lack of sensation and the potential damaging effect of edema, careful attention must be directed to obtaining a congruous splint fit that minimizes pressure and does not obstruct venous return or arterial flow. Straps and splint components may be widened to alleviate undue pressure on underlying soft tissue (Fig. 11-25); splints that apply small areas of three-point pressure or are circumferential in design are contraindicated during the early mobilization of a replanted segment. Careful monitoring of the replant is essential after splint application. An alteration of digital color or increase in edema of the replanted segment necessitates immediate removal of the splint. As the vascular status of the replant becomes less tenuous, its sensitivity to pressure decreases, allowing the use of more conventional splint designs.

TENDON GRAFTS

Tendon grafting involves the bridging of a gap in tendon with an autogenous donor tendon from the same or a separate extremity. Commonly used donor tendons include the palmaris longus, the plantaris, and on occasion a toe extensor. One of the most important criteria for a successful tendon graft procedure is the establishment and maintenance of good passive motion of the disabled segment and adjacent rays. Splinting may be effectively employed for creating and preserving supple digits, both preoperatively and during the postoperative course.

Preoperative splinting should be designed to meet the individual problems presented. If wrist position does not influence passive motion, simple and compound

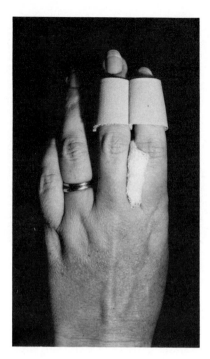

Fig. 11-26. The use of a "finger trapper" facilitates the maintenance of passive motion during the preoperative phase of a tendon graft procedure.

splints such as a short dorsal outrigger, safety pin, wristband with fingernail clips, or a web spacer are usually efficient devices for maximizing passive joint motion. If, however, significant wrist-produced tenodesing of the extrinsic flexor or extensor tendons is present, the wrist must be incorporated into the splint to control its influence at digital levels. Once passive motion is reestablished, the splinting program may be directed to maintenance techniques, which often involve uncomplicated night splinting and a routine exercise program during the day (Fig. 11-26).

The philosophy of postoperative management to which one subscribes dictates the type of splinting program employed after surgical attachment of the tendon graft. Some authors advocate immobilization of the hand for three weeks to promote tendon healing before initiating splinting and conservative therapy, whereas others begin early controlled passive motion in hopes of diminishing scar formation between the sutured graft and its gliding bed. It appears, however, that many of the adhesion-modifying benefits of early controlled motion after primary flexor tendon repair are not applicable to tendon grafting, and results following the application of these techniques to grafts have been disappointing. The splinting programs differ considerably and should not be undertaken without knowledge of the postoperative management plan for each patient and without a thorough understanding of the concepts involved. (See also the section on postoperative splinting of tendon repairs.)

Staged flexor tendon grafts

The general concepts employed in the management of single-stage tendon grafts may be applied to the treatment of two-stage flexor tendon grafting procedures, except that the pregraft time period is expanded to allow the development of a pseudosheath around a flexible tendon implant that is removed at the time of grafting. As with the one-stage grafts, a supple hand is a prerequisite to surgical procedures. Once this is established, a flexible tendon implant is inserted with its distal end anchored to the tendon stub or to bone. Postoperatively the hand and wrist are immobilized in flexion posture for approximately three weeks, during which time the pseudosheath forms, providing a smooth gliding bed for the second-stage autogenous graft. Early splinting may be required to reestablish preoperative passive motion levels. Finger taping, frequent conscientious exercise periods, and individualized splinting are the keys to maintaining good passive motion during the first stage of the postoperative phase.

Once the implant is removed and the tendon graft connected, the two-stage procedure is treated similarly to the single-stage tendon graft (see the following section).

TENDON REPAIRS

Splinting involved in tendon repairs falls into two categories: splints used in the early passive mobilization techniques for flexor tendon repairs in zones one and two and those used to protect or to enhance motion once active motion of the repair has been initiated.

Traditionally tendon repairs have been immobilized from three to five weeks before motion is permitted. However, it has been well demonstrated by Mason (1941) that there is little or no tensile strength at a flexor tendon repair site until it is subjected to stress. Kleinert et al. (1975) and Duran (1978) have developed methods for early passive mobilization of repaired flexor tendons in "no-man's-land" that seem to lessen the effect of amplitude-limiting adhesions on the repaired tendon. The method of Kleinert and colleagues is based on use of antagonistic active extension, whereas Duran advocates passive motion at the interphalangeal joints. Both methods require careful adherence to specific splinting and exercise routines, and neither should be undertaken without a thorough understanding of the concepts involved. Although splints developed to be used with these early mobilization techniques differ in configuration, similarities exist. Each requires a posture of wrist flexion to decrease tension on the repair and some method of eliminating active digital flexion and passive digital extension while permitting periods of limited passive excursion of the flexor tendon repair (Fig. 11-27).

When designing a splint for early passive mobilization, one should consider the effect of integrated motion of the flexor tendons, which to some degree limits independent digital action. Because the index finger and the thumb are considered the only truly independent digits, repair of the long, ring, or small flexor tendons necessitates inclusion of all three digits in the splint.

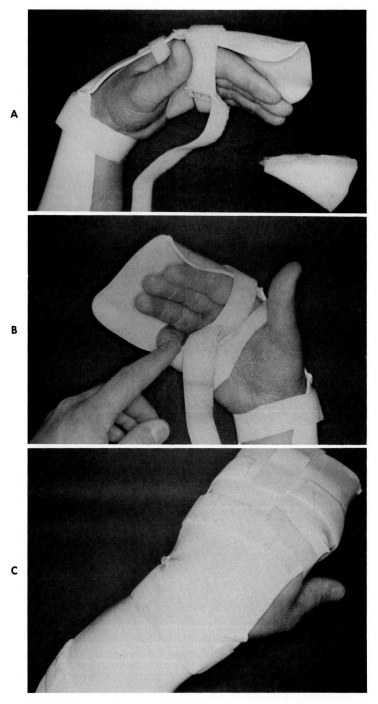

Fig. 11-27. A, A foam wedge that maintains the interphalangeal joints in a posture of slight flexion is removed **(B)** for passive exercise in this splint designed for use with the Duran method of early mobilization of flexor tendon repairs. **C,** Dorsal view of splint.

Repaired flexor or extensor tendons that have been treated with initial immobilization may require a period of protective splinting to prevent undue accidental stress to the repair site between controlled exercise periods. Flexion of the wrist and digital joints decreases tension on flexor repairs; conversely, extensor repairs are protected with extension positioning. It should be remembered, however, that these positions require greater active excursion of the tendon to effect joint motion, and active exercises done in these splints may be less effective than with reverse positioning to increase tension. The patient should thoroughly understand the exercise and splinting programs before being allowed to proceed with an unsupervised course of self-therapy. As tensile strength increases, the protective positioning may be gradually changed and ultimately discarded. If joints that have become stiffened during the period of immobilization do not respond to exercises, mobilization splinting may be required with methods selected that do not impart stress to the tendon repair. Gentle mobilization splinting in a direction that stresses the tendon repair site may be applied concomitant with the initiation of light resistive exercises about six to eight weeks after surgery.

TENDON TRANSFERS

In developing a rehabilitation program for the patient with a partially paralyzed hand who is a candidate for the transference of muscle power, it is imperative that the therapist work closely with the physician to understand the exact deficit and the specific plans for surgical restoration. Postoperatively it is equally important to gain a thorough appreciation of the transfers used, their course, and realistic functional goals. Without this understanding the patient may be subjected to ineffective and unreasonable exercise and splinting programs that will often diminish the benefit of the tendon transfers.

The splinting and exercise program used with tendon transfers may be divided into three chronologic subcategories: (1) preoperative phase, (2) early postoperative phase, and (3) late postoperative phase. Each phase is characterized by distinctly different purposes for exercise and splinting.

It is important that exercise programs be implemented at an early stage in the management of the patient who has developed paralysis secondary to the interruption or disease of a major peripheral nerve. When tendon transfers are anticipated, the strengthening of donor muscles may be helpful, particularly if testing indicates that weakness has developed secondary to disuse. Predictable patterns of paralysis may be seen after median, ulnar, or radial nerve loss, and consultation with the hand surgeon will provide valuable information regarding anticipated functional return, potential tendon transfers, and the therapeutic needs of a specific patient.

To obtain maximum benefit from tendon transfer procedures, a hand must be supple. During the preoperative phase, emphasis is placed on attaining and maintaining maximum passive range of motion of wrist and digital joints. If a hand exhibits restricted passive motion, splints must be designed and fitted to correct the specific joint limitations. However, when full passive motion is present and maintenance of this mobility is the indication for splint application, other types of splints may be considered. Manual muscle test data and active range-of-motion measurements govern the designing of a splint that may be used to prevent the development of joint stiffness while allowing improved functional use of the partially paralyzed hand. Splints employed to prevent deformity from occurring in some of the more common types of peripheral upper extremity paralyses are described in the section of this chapter on peripheral nerve injury.

Early postoperative splinting encompasses three facets: (1) protection of the transfer after dressing removal, (2) correction of stiffness secondary to the immobilization necessitated by surgery, and (3) controlled increase of tension on the transferred musculotendinous unit(s).

Splinting may be used to protect tendon transfer during the earliest stages of mobilization. These splints are designed to decrease tension on the transfer and are used before and during exercise periods and at night (Fig. 11-28). They are usually discarded within the first week of mobilization.

Because of the period of immobilization that is required to promote healing after surgical intervention, adjacent uninvolved joints may become stiff and require splinting measures to regain diminished passive motions. Joints whose stiffness originates from this relatively brief period of immobilization usually respond quickly to splinting efforts and require little more than exercise to maintain motion once it has been regained.

The third reason for employing splinting in the early postoperative phase is to gradually increase the tension on transferred tendons to help stretch any adhesion that may have formed and to allow for the initiation of mechanically advantageous active motion. Careful control of splint traction techniques during this phase may

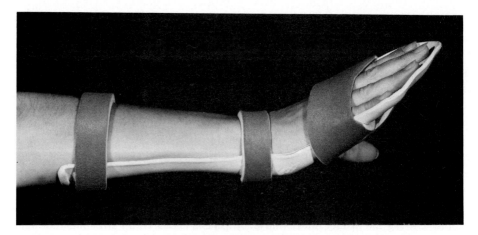

Fig. 11-28. This complex wrist and finger immobilization night splint eliminates tension on an extrinsic transfer that runs dorsal to the wrist axis of rotation.

allow the splinted joints to regain the desired range of motion without the unfavorable reverse deformity that sometimes accompanies tight transfers. Timing of this type of splinting may correspond with the initiation of light resistive exercises and activities.

Altering the position of joints crossed by the specific musculotendinous combination of a given transfer permits an increase or decrease in the tension stress on the tendon. Immobilizing the wrist in a direction opposite to the side in which the tendon transfer was routed will effectively tighten the transfer and maximize its function. An example of this tenodesis effect may be seen in the tension imparted to a donor motor tendon that passes volarly to the wrist axis by placing the wrist in extension. Similarly, a posture of wrist flexion would intensify the pull on the dorsally placed extrinsic donor (Fig. 11-29). In cases of tendon transfers designed to function across multiple digital joints, the splint may be extended distally to position consecutive joints in attitudes that will effectively control tension. As the amplitude and tensile strength increases and active motion of the involved joints improves, the use of splints may be gradually eliminated to permit unassisted use of the transfer.

Splinting in the late postoperative phase involves the conversion of learned substitution patterns by gradually eliminating the mechanically advantageous use of wrist tenodesis and requiring greater excursion of the donor musculotendinous unit(s). The wrist may now be gradually positioned in an attitude opposite to that used in the early postoperative phase with active contraction of the motor tendon replacing the tension imparted by the splint. The concept now is to decrease postural tension on the donor musculotendinous unit and force greater tendon excursion to accomplish segmental motion.

It is important to note that the requirement for splinting during the postopera-

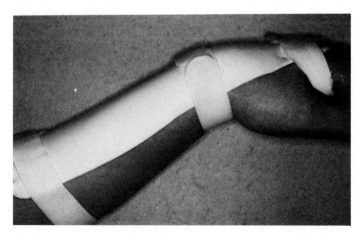

Fig. 11-29. Wrist flexion increases the tension on a dorsally placed extrinsic donor tendon and mechanically facilitates active digital extension.

tive phase of tendon transfers may be extremely variable, depending heavily on the specific transfer procedure used, the expertise of the surgeon, and the inherent adaptability of the patient. Many patients require only initial instruction at the time of dressing removal, readily accommodating to the altered kinetic and kinematic effects of the transfer procedure. This is particularly true in patients whose tendon transfers have been synergistic with wrist flexors used for finger extension and wrist extensors for finger flexion. Others, often with "out-of-phase" transfers, will require considerable assistance in the form of splinting, exercise, and guidance to attain acceptable tendon transfer performance.

TENOLYSIS

Tenolysis involves the surgical freeing of adhesions around a tendon to improve tendon gliding and excursion. Active range-of-motion exercises and splinting are usually initiated within the first 24-hour period after surgery.

A tenolysis program employs splinting to achieve and maintain passive motion preoperatively and to maintain passive range of motion postoperatively. Preoperative splints are designed to correct specific joint limitations and may be used at night to sustain passive motion once it has been achieved. The most common types of splints used to augment postoperative motion are of the simple and compound classifications. Alternation of both flexion and extension splints may be required, and, despite the involvement of extrinsic tendons, the need to immobilize the wrist is unusual. However, if the patient consistently assumes a protective wrist posture that is unfavorable to use of maximum tendon amplitude, a complex splint that favorably positions the wrist as an adjunctive measure to digital mobilization should be applied. For instance, after flexor tenolysis, if the patient uses an inefficient wrist flexion posture when flexing the digits, a complex splint that immobilizes the wrist in extension will encourage greater flexor tendon excursion.

Because active motion is paramount after a tenolysis procedure, splint wearing times must be interspersed with frequent exercise periods. Depending on individual circumstances, patients are often instructed to exercise 15 minutes of every hour and to alternate splints every 1 to 2 hours during the day. In addition, patients are usually instructed to sleep in the splint, which imparts either dynamic or static positioning to correct problem motion. Exercise and splinting programs must be continuously reevaluated and adapted as changes in motion status occur. As active motion improves, the splinting program may be gradually curtailed to permit progressively longer durations of unassisted functional hand use. Night splinting is continued until the patient is able to consistently maintain active passive motion through exercise alone.

SUMMARY

From these sections one can see that special problems relating to hand injury and disease and the appropriate surgical management of these conditions present somewhat predictable splinting requirements. Although broad generalization with regard to the splinting of these problems can be offered, it is obvious that wide variations occur in the clinical presentation of each problem and its therapeutic approach. Armed with an appreciation of the potential peculiarities of each of these general categories, one can become familiarized with the individual circumstances and subsequently initiate the most applicable splinting and exercise program.

CHAPTER 12

Analysis of splints

It is apparent that most of the mistakes made in hand splinting are caused by inattention to detail. For the most part, the types of splints are chosen correctly according to the circumstances presented but fail to be effective because of relatively minor design or adjustment factors that cause discomfort, functional ineffectiveness, or poor appearance. Each splint fitted on a patient must be thoroughly evaluated according to the principles of design, construction, fit, and mechanics. Failure to do so may not only produce improper results but may actually cause additional deformity.

The purpose of this chapter is to provide the reader with an opportunity to apply the theoretical material presented in the previous chapters and to allow for immediate independent assessment through self-evaluation techniques. Acknowledging that there can be no substitute for actual experiential learning, it is hoped that this chapter will initiate, facilitate, and strengthen sound analytical thinking in regard to splint design and fabrication.

On the following pages illustrations of improperly constructed splints are presented and analyzed according to classification, purpose of application, clinical problems, and solutions to the problems. The splints, although generally constructed correctly, incorporate one or more common mistakes that clinically produce diminished results. The reader is asked to assess these illustrations using the information in the preceding chapters of this book as a theoretical framework. Comparison of one's results with those presented here will provide a standard for self-evaluation.

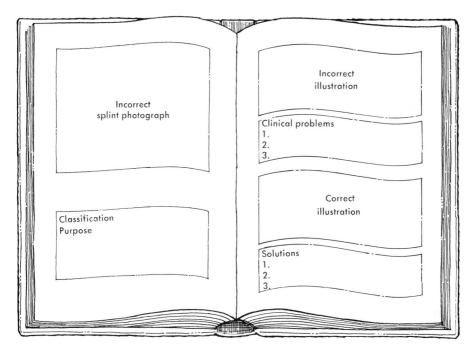

Fig. 12-1. Each splint analysis unit is presented in a consistent order: incorrect splint photograph, classification and purpose, incorrect drawing, clinical problems, corrected drawing, and solutions to clinical problems.

So that the reader may more readily adapt this chapter to a personal level of expertise, the format of splint illustrations and their accompanying assessments is presented consistently (Fig. 12-1). By blocking out selected sections, for example, "clinical problems" and "solutions" or "classification" and "purpose(s)," throughout the chapter (Figs. 12-2 to 12-19), the amount of background information given about each splint illustrated may be varied, making analysis more or less difficult. For example, the novice may choose not to block any of the sections, allowing open comparison of the classification, purposes, problems, and solutions of each example, whereas someone with intermediate experience may identify the blocked-out problems and solutions knowing only the classification and purpose of application of the splints. Finally, the blocking of all four sections and the "incorrect/correct" drawings requires the reader to independently identify the classification, purposes, problems, and solutions of each splint picture. Use of the splint checkout form (Appendix C) may be helpful in providing an organizational basis for splint analysis. For immediate feedback, we recommend that readers compare their conclusions regarding the specific illustration they have analyzed before moving on to the next splint picture. Red indicates areas of changes in the correct drawings.   *Text continued on p. 278.*

Fig. 12-2

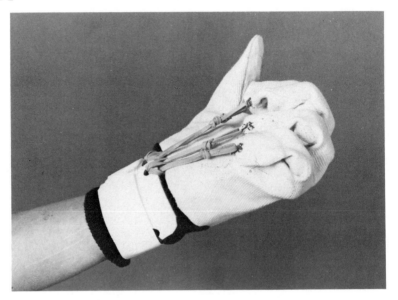

Classification
Simple finger flexion splint
Purpose
To flex the metacarpophalangeal and interphalangeal joints of the fingers.

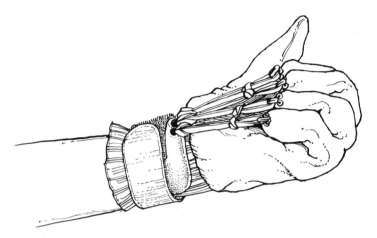

Clinical problems

1. The traction does not adequately affect the stiffer metacarpophalangeal joints.
2. The glove decreases sensory feedback, is bulky and hot, and retains moisture and dirt.

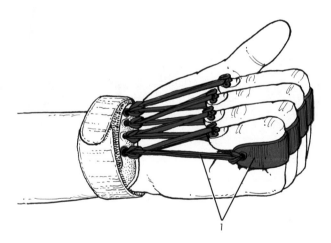

Solutions

1. Add dynamic traction to individual joints such as finger cuff for metacarpophalangeal flexion, fingernail clip for proximal interphalangeal flexion, or glove rubber band for distal interphalangeal flexion.
2. A wrist cock-up with volar outrigger may be necessary to provide a 90-degree angle of pull of the traction device (see Fig. 12-13).

Fig. 12-3

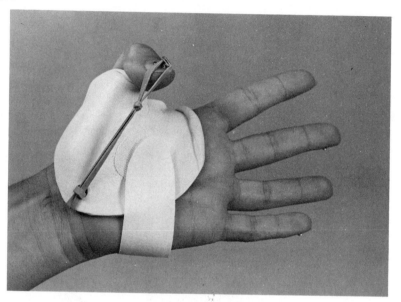

Classification
Compound thumb IP flexion splint
Purposes
1. To flex the interphalangeal joint of the thumb.
2. To maintain the thumb web space.

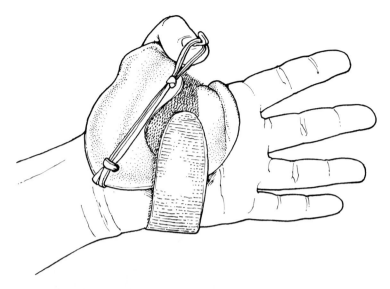

Clinical problems
1. Because the angle of the dynamic traction is not perpendicular to the axis of rotation of the interphalangeal joint, unequal stress is applied to the collateral ligaments and may result in ulnar collateral ligament damage.
2. The distal end of the splint inhibits index and long metacarpophalangeal flexion.

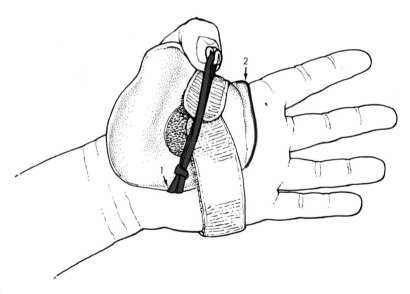

Solutions
1. Adjust the elastic traction to provide a perpendicular angle of approach to the interphalangeal joint axis of rotation.
2. Roll the distal edge of the splint proximally. It should not extend beyond the distal palmar flexion crease.

Fig. 12-4

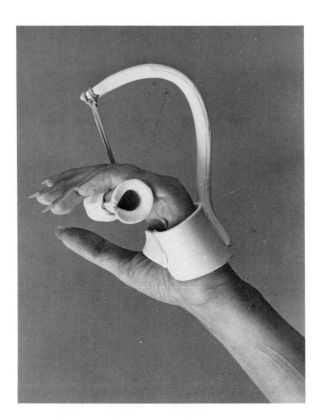

Classification
Simple MP extension splint
Purpose
To extend the metacarpophalangeal joints.

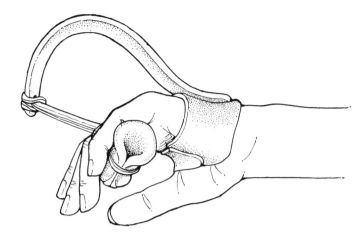

Clinical problems
1. The distal aspect of the dorsal metacarpal bar is causing pressure on dorsum of hand.
2. Flexion of ring and small proximal interphalangeal joints is limited by volar lumbrical bar.
3. The transverse arch is not supported at the phalangeal level.
4. Second to fifth metacarpophalangeal joints are mobilized in unison.
5. The 60-degree angle of elastic traction to proximal phalanges causes the volar phalangeal bar to slip distally.

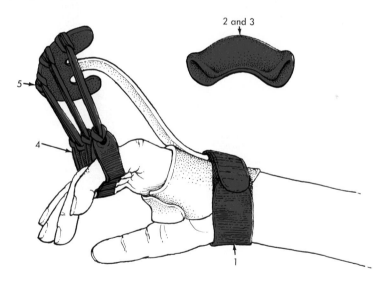

Solutions
1. Add a wrist strap to the proximal aspect of the dorsal metacarpal bar.
2. Adjust the phalangeal bar to allow for differences in the lengths of the digital rays.
3. Adjust the phalangeal bar to support the transverse arch at the proximal phalangeal level.
4. Add individual metacarpophalangeal extension finger cuffs.
5. Design and adjust the extension outrigger to provide a 90-degree pull of the elastic traction to proximal phalanges that also provides a perpendicular force to the sagittal axis of rotation of each joint. (NOTE: Use either 2 and 3; or 4.)

Fig. 12-5

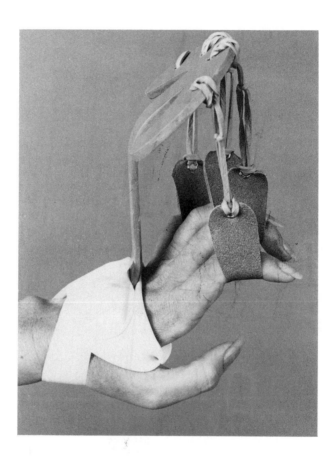

Classification
Simple finger extension splint
Purpose
To extend the proximal interphalangeal joints.

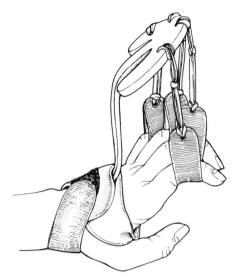

Clinical problems

1. The more mobile metacarpophalangeal joints are hyperextended.
2. The angle of elastic traction to the proximal phalanges enhances metacarpophalangeal joint hyperextension.
3. The finger cuffs prevent full interphalangeal joint flexion.
4. The uncovered Velcro hook fastener is abrasive to clothing.

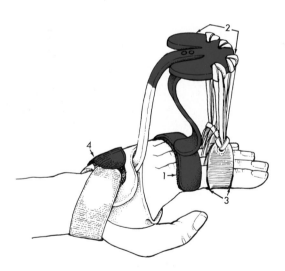

Solutions

1. Add a lumbrical bar to prevent metacarpophalangeal hypertension. NOTE: Classification changes to compound proximal interphalangeal extension splint.
2. Adjust outrigger to provide a 90-degree angle of the elastic traction to middle phalanges.
3. Trim the proximal and distal edges of the finger cuffs to interphalangeal joint flexion.
4. Lengthen the wrist strap to provide full closure.

Fig. 12-6

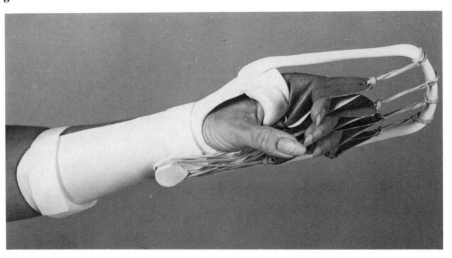

Classification
Complex MP flexion/PIP extension splint
Purposes
1. To flex the metacarpophalangeal joints.
2. To extend the proximal interphalangeal joints.
3. To immobilize the wrist joint.

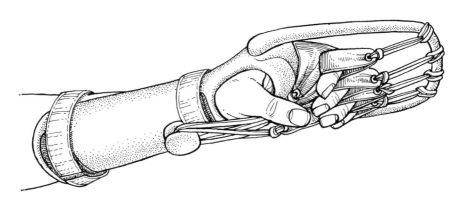

Clinical problems
1. The antagonistic elastic traction on consecutive joints results in diminished flexion and extension forces.
2. The distal end of the splint inhibits flexion of the metacarpophalangeal joints.
3. The acute angle of approach of elastic flexion traction to the proximal phalanges results in metacarpophalangeal joint compression.
4. The angle of elastic extension traction to the middle phalanges results in diminished rotational force and may cause metacarpophalangeal hyperextension.
5. The finger cuffs inhibit interphalangeal joint flexion.
6. The ends of the straps have sharp corners.

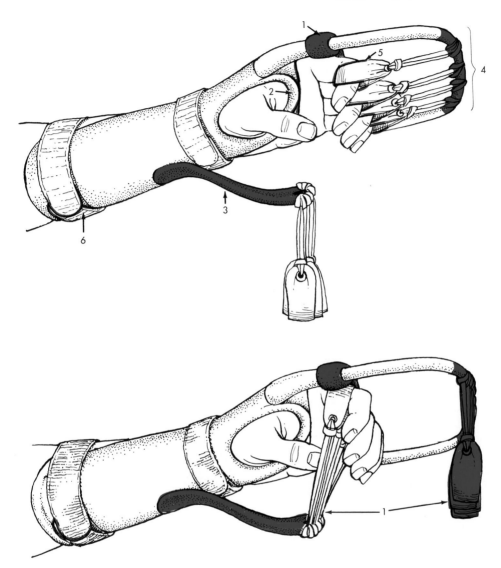

Solutions
1. If the metacarpophalangeal joints exhibit full flexion, add an immobile lumbrical bar to stabilize the proximal phalanges and to prevent hyperextension. If the metacarpophalangeal joints lack flexion, separate wearing times for metacarpophalangeal flexion and proximal interphalangeal extension, and add a lumbrical bar to prevent metacarpophalangeal hyperextension while in the extension cuffs.
2. Adjust the distal end of the splint to be proximal to the distal palmar flexion crease.
3. Add a volar outrigger to provide a 90-degree angle of approach of the elastic traction to the proximal phalanges.
4. Adjust the outrigger to provide a 90-degree angle of approach of the elastic traction to the middle phalanges.
5. Contour the extension finger cuffs.
6. Round the ends of the straps.

Fig. 12-7

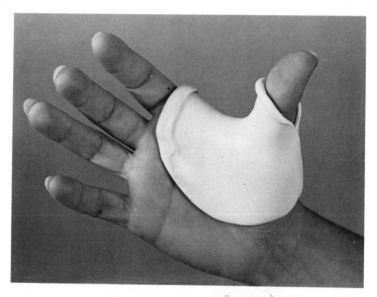

Classification
Simple thumb CMC extension/abduction splint
Purpose
To increase or maintain the thumb web space.

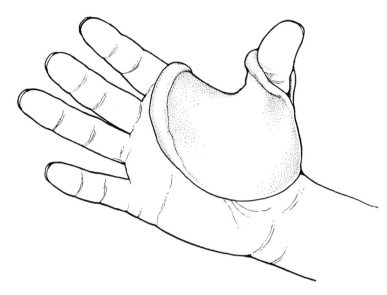

Clinical problems
1. Flexion of the index and long metacarpophalangeal joints is inhibited by the distal end of the splint.
2. Thumb interphalangeal flexion is limited by the distal end of the thumb post.
3. Distal migration of the splint results in application of the rotational force to the proximal phalanx of the thumb with potential stretching of the metacarpophalangeal ulnar collateral ligament.

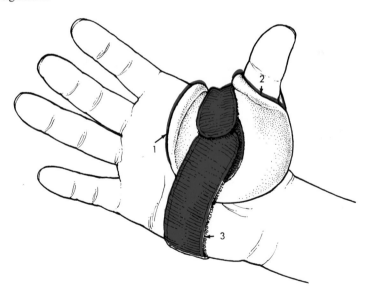

Solutions
1. Adjust the distal edge of the splint to end proximal to the distal palmar flexion crease.
2. Adjust the distal edge of the thumb post to the end proximal to the flexion crease of the thumb interphalangeal joint.
3. Add a strap for stabilization of the splint in the web space.

Fig. 12-8

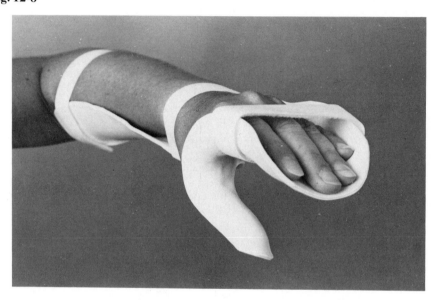

Classification
Complex finger and thumb immobilization splint
Purposes
1. To immobilize the metacarpophalangeal and interphalangeal joints in slight flexion.
2. To immobilize the thumb in abduction.
3. To maintain the thumb web space.
4. To immobilize the wrist joint in slight extension.

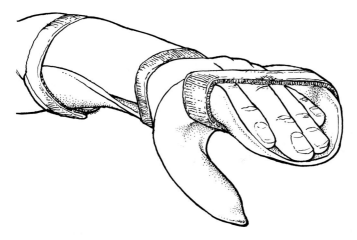

Clinical problems
1. Elbow flexion is limited by the proximal end of the splint.
2. The transverse arch is not supported at the phalangeal level.
3. The high edges of the finger pan prevent finger positioning by the distal strap.
4. The distal end of the thumb post is too long.

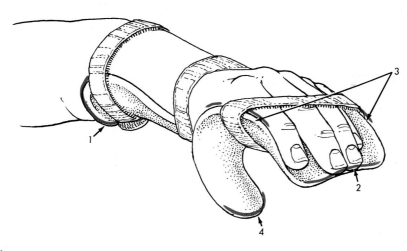

Solutions
1. Shorten the forearm trough to two thirds of "inside elbow" length and flange the proximal end.
2. Continue the transverse arch the length of the finger pan.
3. Decrease the lateral and medial borders to provide continuous contact of the strap across the dorsal aspect of the fingers.
4. Decrease the distal length of the thumb post.

Fig. 12-9

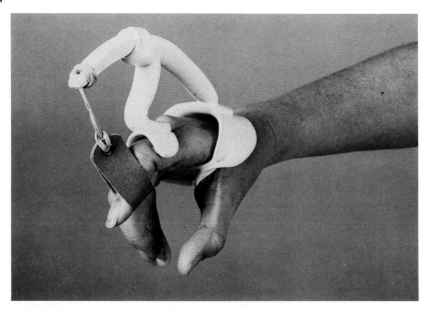

Classification
Compound PIP extension splint
Purpose
To extend the index proximal interphalangeal joint.

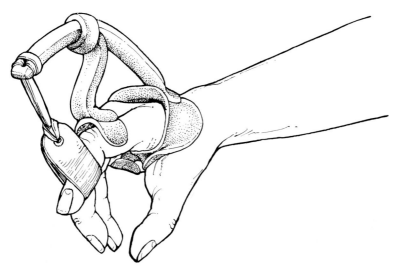

Clinical problems
1. The dorsal and palmar metacarpal bars are loose and allow the outrigger to rotate.
2. The proximal edge of the lumbrical bar creates pressure on the dorsum of the proximal phalanx.
3. The angle of the elastic traction to the middle phalanx diminishes the magnitude of the rotational force and compresses the proximal interphalangeal joint surfaces.
4. The finger cuff inhibits interphalangeal joint flexion.

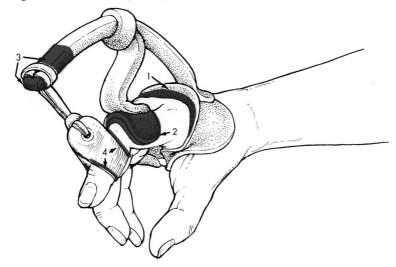

Solutions
1. Adjust the dorsal and palmar metacarpal bars to provide continuous circumferential contact.
2. Adjust the lumbrical bar to provide equal pressure on the dorsum of the phalanx. To further disseminate pressure, add foam padding to the volar aspect of the lumbrical bar.
3. Adjust the outrigger to provide a 90-degree angle of elastic traction to the middle phalanx. This traction should also be perpendicular to the axis of joint rotation.
4. Trim the proximal and distal edges of the finger cuff.

Fig. 12-10

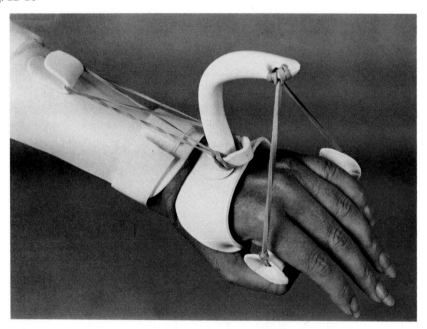

Classification
Simple wrist and MP extension splint
Purposes
1. To extend the wrist.
2. To extend the metacarpophalangeal joints.

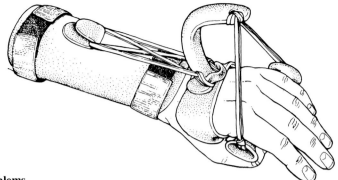

Clinical problems

1. Distal migration of the forearm trough causes pressure on the dorsum of the wrist and on the ulnar styloid process.
2. The 20-degree angle of elastic wrist traction to the metacarpals creates joint compression at the carpal level.
3. The ring and small proximal interphalangeal joint flexion is limited by the volar phalangeal bar.
4. The transverse arch is not supported at the phalangeal level.
5. The metacarpophalangeal joints are mobilized in unison.
6. The angle of approach of elastic traction to the proximal phalanges results in decreased magnitude of the rotational force.
7. The Velcro hook is abrasive to clothing, and the strap corners are sharp.

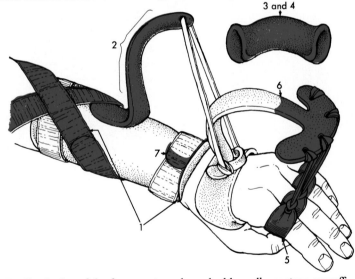

Solutions

1. Flange the distal edge of the forearm trough, and add an elbow strap or cuff.
2. Add a dorsal outrigger to provide a 90-degree pull of the elastic traction to metacarpals.
3. Adjust the phalangeal bar to allow for differences in longitudinal lengths of digital rays.
4. Revise the phalangeal bar to support the transverse arch at the proximal phalangeal level.
5. Add individual metacarpophalangeal extension finger cuffs.
6. Adjust the outrigger to provide a 90-degree angle of the elastic traction to the proximal phalanges. The traction devices should also be perpendicular to the sagittal axis of rotation of each metacarpalphalangeal joint.
7. Round the strap corners, and lengthen the straps to complete closure.
   (NOTE: Use either 3 and 4, or 5.)

Fig. 12-11

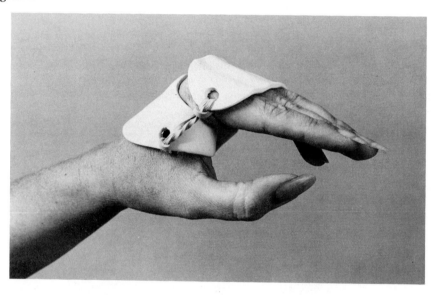

Classification
Simple MP flexion splint
Purpose
To flex the metacarpophalangeal joints.

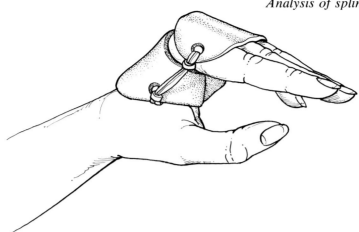

Clinical problems
1. Pressure exists in the thumb web space from the palmar metacarpal bar.
2. The dorsal lumbrical bar migrates proximally.
3. The metacarpal bars migrate distally.
4. The acute angle of approach of elastic traction to the proximal phalanges results in diminished rotational force on the metacarpophalangeal joints.
5. The metacarpophalangeal joints are mobilized in unison.

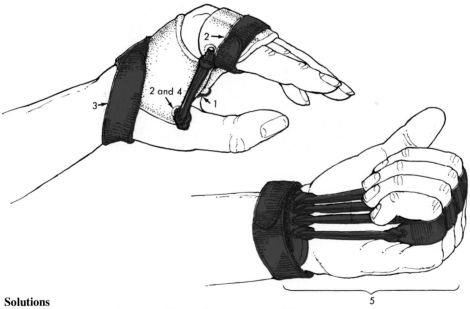

Solutions
1. Flange the proximal aspect of the palmar metacarpal bar edge.
2. Correct the angle of rotational traction to a perpendicular pull, and add a phalangeal strap.
3. Add a wrist strap.
4. Design the splint to provide a 90-degree angle of the elastic traction to proximal phalanges, which is also perpendicular to the axis of sagittal rotation.
5. Use either a wristband with metacarpophalangeal flexion cuffs or a simple wrist immobilization splint with volar outrigger (Fig. 12-14) instead of the splint illustrated.

Fig. 12-12

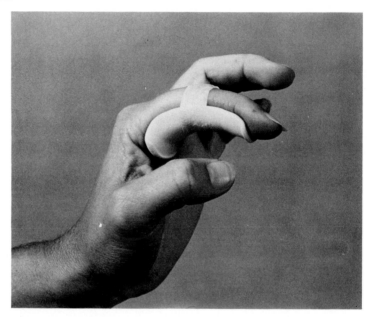

Classification
Simple PIP flexion block splint
Purpose
To prevent index proximal interphalangeal joint flexion beyond 30 degrees.

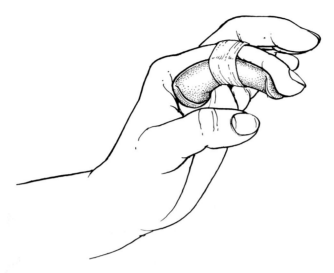

Clinical problem
The distal end of the splint limits distal interphalangeal joint flexion.

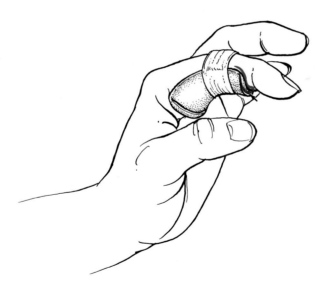

Solution
Shorten the distal splint edge to end proximal to the distal interphalangeal joint flexion crease.

Fig. 12-13

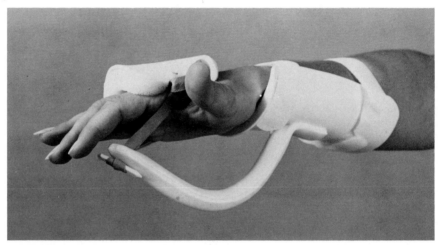

Classification
Simple wrist flexion splint
Purpose
To flex the wrist.

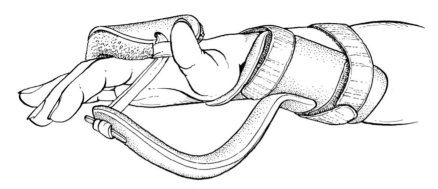

Clinical problems
1. The distal aspect of the forearm trough is too wide.
2. The lateral and medial borders of the dorsal metacarpal cuff may cause pressure areas on the dorsum of the hand.
3. The dorsal metacarpal cuff migrates distally.
4. The angle of approach of the elastic traction to the metacarpals diminishes the magnitude of the rotational force.
5. Pressure exists under the proximal strap.

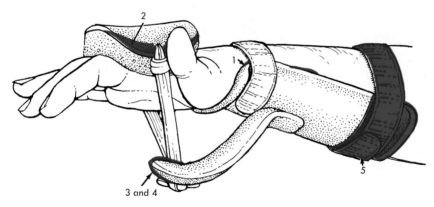

Solutions
1. Decrease the radial border to half the width of the forearm.
2. Widen the dorsal metacarpal cuff.
3 and 4. Adjust the outrigger to provide a 90-degree angle of the elastic traction to the metacarpals.
5. Lengthen the forearm trough and move the strap proximally.

Fig. 12-14

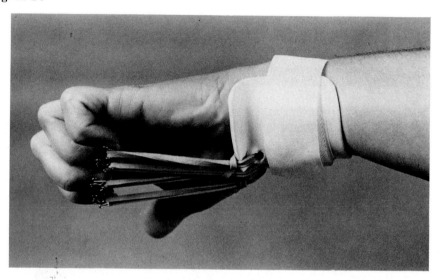

Classification
Simple finger flexion splint
Purpose
To flex the metacarpophalangeal joints.

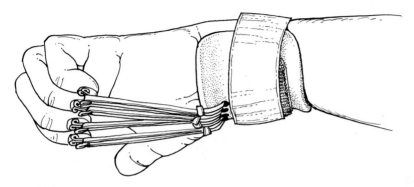

Clinical problem
Because of the difference in the mobility of the metacarpophalangeal and interphalangeal
joints, the magnitude of the traction is dissipated at the level of the interphalangeal joints.

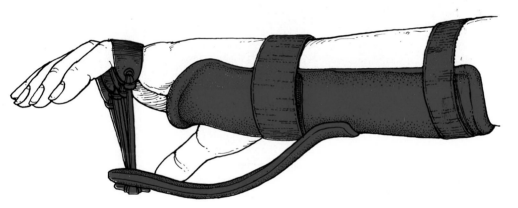

Solution
Change the design of the splint to a volar wrist cock-up with an outrigger with individual
metacarpophalangeal flexion cuffs. NOTE: Classification changes to complex metacarpophalangeal flexion splint.

Fig. 12-15

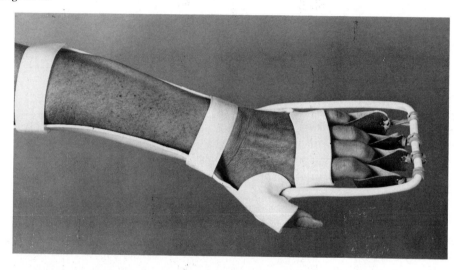

Classification
Compound complex PIP extension splint with thumb CMC and MP immobilization
Purposes
1. To extend the proximal interphalangeal joints.
2. To immobilize the thumb carpometacarpal and metacarpophalangeal joints.
3. To immobilize the wrist joint.

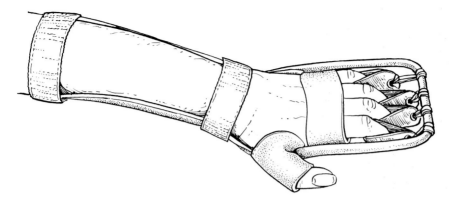

Clinical problems
1. The ulnar aspect of the forearm trough is causing pressure on the ulnar border of the forearm.
2. Thumb interphalangeal flexion is limited by the distal edge of the thumb post.
3. The metacarpophalangeal joints are hyperextended.
4. The angle of approach of elastic traction to the middle phalanges causes the finger cuffs to migrate distally.
5. The outrigger is too short to allow satisfactory application of the elastic traction.
6. The radial aspect of the wrist bar is not fitted closely.

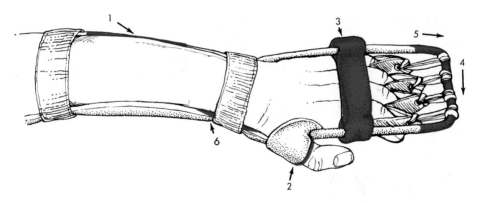

Solutions
1. Refit the ulnar forearm trough to decrease the pressure on the ulnar border of the forearm.
2. Roll the distal edge of the thumb post proximal to the interphalangeal joint flexion crease.
3. Fit the lumbrical bar to prevent metacarpophalangeal hyperextension and move it distally to more equally cover the proximal phalanges and to allow for the differences in the lengths of the longitudinal rays.
4. Adjust the outrigger to provide a 90-degree angle of approach of the elastic traction to the middle phalanges.
5. Lengthen the outrigger or attach rubber bands on the lumbrical bar with a fulcrum over the outrigger.
6. Improve the contour of the radial wrist bar to the wrist.

Fig. 12-16

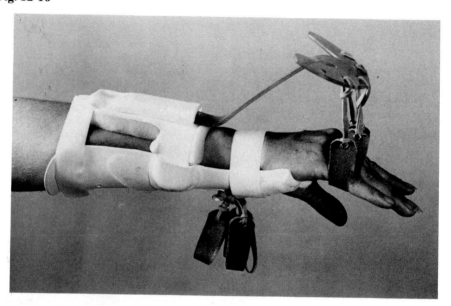

Classification
Complex MP extension/flexion splint
Purposes
1. To extend the metacarpophalangeal joints.
2. To flex the metacarpophalangeal joints.
3. To immobilize the wrist.

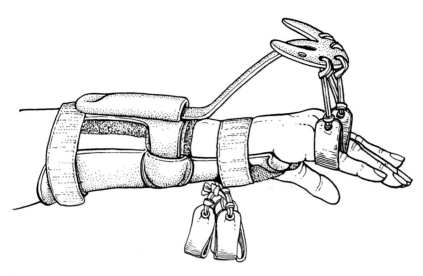

Clinical problems
1. The wrist is not fully immobilized.
2. The outrigger does not provide a rigid basis of attachment for the traction devices.
3. The angle of approach of the elastic traction to the proximal phalanges causes the finger cuffs to cut into the finger webs and decrease the magnitude of the rotational force.
4. It is possible that the angle of pull of the flexion elastic traction to proximal phalanges is incorrect.

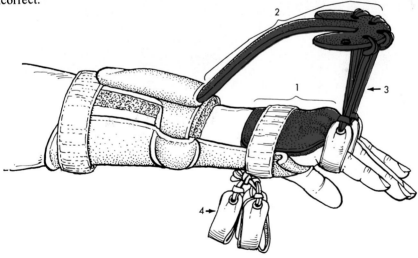

Solutions
1. Add a dorsometacarpal strap or cuff to prevent wrist extension.
2. Construct the outrigger from a stronger material.
3. Adjust the outrigger to provide a 90-degree angle of approach of elastic traction to the proximal phalanges.
4. If the angle of the flexion traction is incorrect, add a volar outrigger, and adjust to allow a 90-degree angle of the dynamic assists to the proximal phalanges.

Fig. 12-17

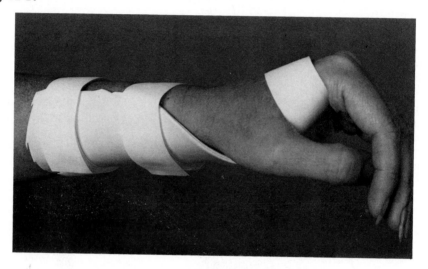

Classification
Simple wrist immobilization splint
Purpose
To immobilize the wrist.

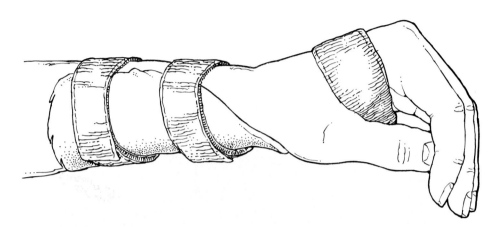

Clinical problems

1. The proximal edge of the splint causes pressure on the forearm.
2. The wrist is not fully immobilized.
3. The strap in the thumb web space causes discomfort.
4. The appearance of the splint is poor.

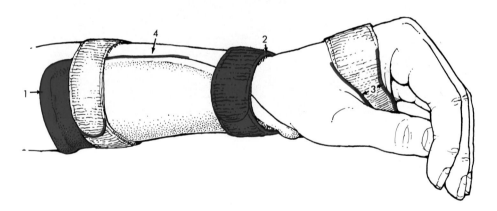

Solutions

1. Increase the length of forearm trough to two thirds the length of the forearm, and flange the proximal end.
2. Position the wrist strap distal to the ulnar styloid process.
3. Contour the distal edge of the strap in the thumb web space.
4. Cut splint edges smoothly, and round the strap ends.

Fig. 12-18

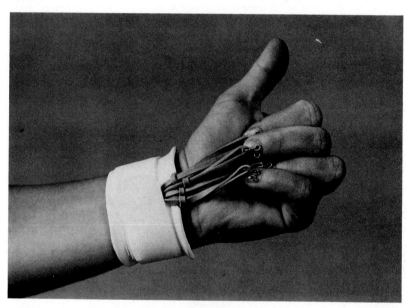

Classification
Simple finger flexion splint
Purpose
To flex the fingers.

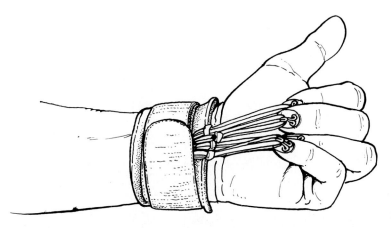

Clinical problem
The single hole causes fingers to "bunch" when flexed simultaneously.

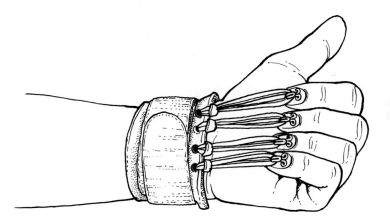

Solution
Design the splint to allow the dynamic traction to arise from three or four separate, slightly radial holes.

Fig. 12-19

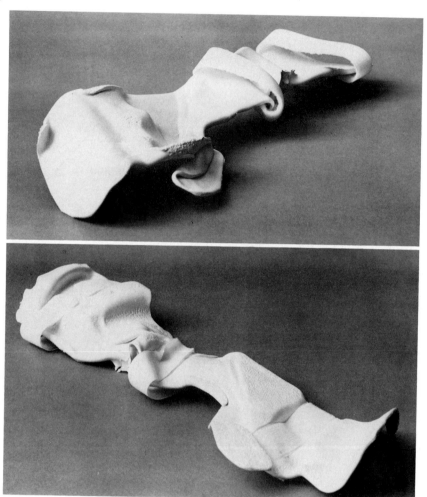

Classification
Complex finger/thumb immobilization splint
Purposes
1. To immobilize the finger metacarpophalangeal and interphalangeal joints in slight flexion.
2. To immobilize the thumb in abduction.
3. To maintain the thumb web space.
4. To immobilize the wrist joint in slight extension.

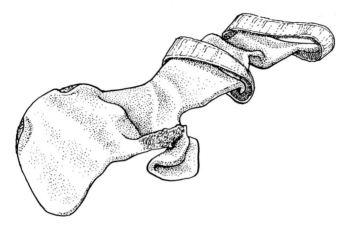

Clinical problem
The splint was left in a closed car on a hot day, which resulted in numerous fit problems.

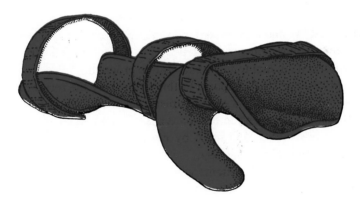

Solution
Start over.

CHAPTER 13

Splinting in a hand surgical practice

During the past fifty years there has been increasing recognition of the role that splinting techniques may play in the reconstruction and rehabilitation of the hand that has become disabled because of congenital defects, disease, or injury. Bunnell's work in the 1940s contributed immensely to the expansion of splinting knowledge, and currently most hand surgeons employ some form of splinting.

The purpose of this chapter is to provide a retrospective statistical analysis of splints used in a large two-physician practice devoted exclusively to the treatment of the entire spectrum of pathologic conditions of the hand and upper extremity. The study encompassed a twelve-month period and included the following specific areas of examination:

1. Type of splint
2. Purpose of application
3. Joints splinted
4. Patient status
5. Diagnosis
6. Type of surgery

It is hoped that the findings presented in this chapter will provide some insight into the splinting requirements of a practice in which splinting is strongly emphasized as an important adjunct to the rehabilitative program.

It should be realized that all splints in this study were the result of direct consultation between the physicians and therapists regarding each patient's individual requirements. With the exception of two types of commercial splints, all splints were designed, constructed, and fitted by either of two registered occupational therapists specializing in hand therapy.

The medical records of all patients who received splints during the year 1977 were reviewed, and data were recorded according to the six previously mentioned categories. Frequency distributions were employed to more clearly identify population trends within the categories.

STATISTICS
Splint types

It was found that during 1977, a total of 1264 hand splints were fitted on 536 patients, an average of 2.4 splints per patient. The splint types ranged from uncomplicated inexpensive devices such as surgical glove bands to sophisticated appliances that provided alternate flexion/extension capabilities. A frequency distribution (Table 2) reveals that, although there were forty-one different types of splints identified, five splint types accounted for more than 50% of the total number constructed (Fig. 13-1): (1) wristband with fingernail clip, (2) cylinder cast, (3) short dorsal outrigger with lumbrical bar, (4) glove rubber band, and (5) safety pin.

It is interesting that, of these five most frequently used splints, with the exception of the short dorsal outrigger, which is a compound splint, all are simple cate-

Table 2. Types of splints*

Splint	Number of splints	Purpose	Joint(s)
Wrist cuff with fingernail clips	166	M	MP, PIP, DIP
Cylinder cast	139	M	PIP
Short dorsal outrigger with lumbrical bar	137	M	PIP
Glove rubber band	123	M	PIP, DIP
Bunnell safety pin	121	M	PIP
Gutter splint, mallet finger splint	106	I	
Thumb web spacer	98	M	T-CMC
Wrist cock-up	53	I	
Static wrist with static thumb abduction	34	I	
Joint jack	26	M	PIP
MP flexion block	26	M-15, I-11	PIP-15
Wristband with MP flexion cuffs	21	M	MP
St. Louis wedge (Weeks)	19	I	
Metacarpophalangeal flexion/extension	17	M	MP
Wrist cock-up with fingernail clips	15	M	MP, PIP, DIP
Protective splint	15	I	
Resting pan	14	I	
Waist cock-up with MP flexion cuffs	14	M	MP
Lone dorsal outrigger with lumbrical bar	14	M	PIP
Metacarpal support	12	I	
Wynn Parry ulnar or ulnar and median nerve	10	C	MP
Distal interphalangeal minioutrigger	10	M	DIP
Dynamic wrist flexion or extension	9	M	W
Short opponens	9	I	
Webbing strap	8	M	PIP
Safe position (Michigan burn)	8	I	
Thumb mobilization splints (CMC, MP, IP)	7	M	CMC, MP, IP
Short dorsal outrigger	7	M	MP
Wrist cock-up with volar outrigger	3	M	MP, PIP, DIP
Long dorsal outrigger	2	M	MP
Wristband with thumb metacarpophalangeal flexion cuff	2	M	T-MP
Duke Velcro finger flexion	3	M	MP, PIP, DIP
Various designs (nine types)	16	M-11, I-5	PIP-5, T-2, W-1, M-3

*M, Mobilize; I, immobilize; C, control; MP, metacarpophalangeal joint; PIP, proximal interphalangeal joint; DIP, distal interphalangeal joint; T, thumb; CMC, carpometacarpal joint; W, wrist.

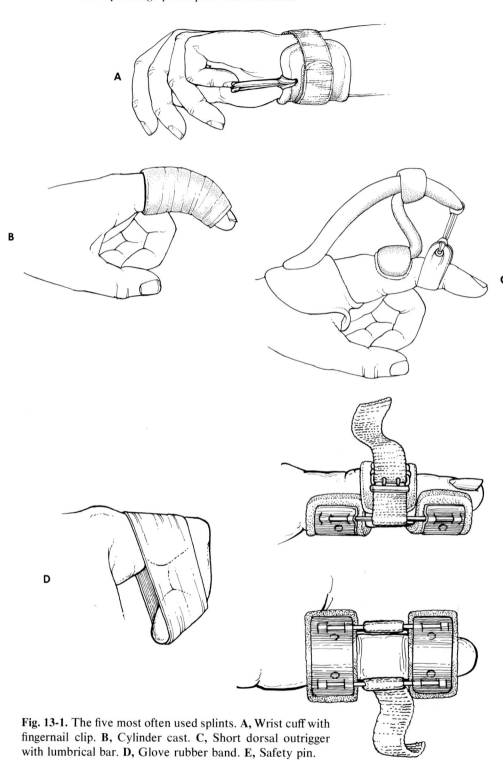

Fig. 13-1. The five most often used splints. **A,** Wrist cuff with fingernail clip. **B,** Cylinder cast. **C,** Short dorsal outrigger with lumbrical bar. **D,** Glove rubber band. **E,** Safety pin.

gory splints. A complex splint with secondary wrist immobilization is not found until approximately the twenty-fifth percentile level. This would corroborate the clinical impression that the majority of hand splints are small and simple rather than the large complicated devices so frequently associated with hand splinting practices.

Purpose of application

Splints designed to deal with joint stiffness (simple and compound) considerably outweighed those prepared for range of motion limitations secondary to tendinous adhesions (complex). It should also be noted that all five most frequently used splints are designed to mobilize joints, and four of the five directly influence the interphalangeal joints. The fifth (wristband with fingernail clip) flexes the metacarpophalangeal joint in addition to the interphalangeal joints.

On further analysis it is found that 76.6% of all the splints fitted in 1977 were designed to mobilize digital segments, 22.6% were fitted for immobilization purposes, and 0.8% were constructed to supply control (Wynn Parry splints for paralysis of the ulnar and of median nerves). If the patient population had included more individuals with spinal cord and upper motor neuron lesions, the number of control splints would certainly have been greater. Of the finger mobilization splints (excluding wrist and thumb), 46% were designed to increase flexion motion, and 54% augmented finger extension.

Joints splinted

Of the total number of mobilization and control splints fitted in this study, 47.6% were designed specifically to enhance proximal interphalangeal joint motion, whereas 79.3% of the splints either influenced the proximal interphalangeal joint directly or acted on it in combination with other joints (Table 3). The metacarpophalangeal joint was mobilized alone or with other joints in slightly more

Table 3. Focus of mobilization and control splints

Joint	Number of splints	Percent of total	
Proximal interphalangeal	465	47.6	
Metacarpophalangeal and proximal and distal interphalangeal	187	19.1	79.3
Proximal and distal interphalangeal	123	12.6	
Thumb carpometacarpal	98	10.0	
Metacarpophalangeal	74	7.6	
Wrist	10	1.0	
Distal interphalangeal	10	1.0	
Thumb carpometacarpal, metacarpophalangeal, and interphalangeal	9	0.9	
Thumb metacarpophalangeal	2	0.2	

than one fourth (26.7%) of the mobilization or control splints. Approximately one third of the splints directly or indirectly affected the distal interphalangeal joint.

It is also of interest that, although wrists were incorporated in more than one sixth of the total number of splints applied in 1977, only 9 (4%) of these splints were oriented toward mobilization of the wrist itself. The remainder were fitted for immobilization purposes as either simple wrist immobilization splints or as complex splints with secondary wrist immobilization.

Splinting and surgical intervention

Of the total number of splints constructed, 12% were fitted during the preoperative phase of treatment and were designed to maintain or increase passive and active range of motion, 78% were fitted postoperatively, and the remaining 10% were fitted to patients who did not require surgery.

Diagnoses

Almost 83% of the patients who required no surgery were diagnosed as having arthrofibrosis. Tendon, ligament, and other soft tissue injuries that did not necessitate surgical intervention but required splinting collectively amounted to slightly more than 13% (Table 4).

Almost a third of the patients (32.2%) who required surgery and splinting suffered from tendon lacerations or avulsions. The second most frequent injury in the

Table 4. Diagnosis of patients who required splinting

Surgery	Percent of patients requiring surgery	No surgery	Percent patients not requiring surgery
Tendon: laceration, avulsion	32.2	Arthrofibrosis	82.6
Bone: fracture, dislocation, subluxation	15.8	Tendon, partial laceration inflammation	6.6
Nerve: laceration, avulsion	12.1	Ligament, soft tissue injury	6.6
Amputation	8.8	Nerve contusion	1.8
Rheumatoid arthritis	7.5	Burn	1.2
Ligament: avulsion, crush, soft tissue injury	7.4	Tumor	0.6
Stenosing tenosynovitis	4.3	Congenital	0.6
Skin: contracture, laceration	3.4		100.0
Tumor	3.3		
Congenital anomalies	1.5		
Artery: laceration	1.0		
Replantation	0.5		
Late ischemic miositis	0.6		
Miscellaneous	1.6		
	100.0		

surgical group encompassed fractures, dislocations, and subluxations (15.8%). Rheumatoid arthritis ranked as the fifth most common diagnosis, requiring a combination of both surgery and rehabilitative splints.

Surgical procedures

The number of patients who required splinting before or after tenolysis or capsulotomy was double that of any other surgical procedure. Tendon repair, arthroplasty, open reduction, tendon transfers, ligamentous repair, and skin grafting also were frequent surgical procedures that necessitated preoperative or postoperative splinting techniques.

SUMMARY

It can be seen from these statistical reviews that hand splinting was an extremely important part of the management of the patients with pathologic hand conditions in this study. Most patients required at least two splints, and simple, easily prepared splints were most commonly used. Splints designed to mobilize stiffened digital joints were the most frequently employed, and the proximal interphalangeal joint was clearly the area of the most problems. Particularly, it was found that the use of splints for the mobilization of joints in the postoperative period was often required and that tenolyses and capsulotomy were the most common surgical procedures lending to splint application.

Although hand splint philosophies and clinical application will vary considerably from practice to practice, this analysis of a particular rehabilitation-oriented hand surgical practice may provide some helpful insight into the splinting potential in similar situations.

APPENDIX A

Mathematic equations for Chapter 3

Fig. 3-11:

$$F \times FA = R \times RA$$
$$F \times 3 = 0.9 \times 2.5$$
$$F \times 3 = 2.25$$
$$F = 0.75$$

$$F \times 5 = 0.9 \times 2.5$$
$$F \times 5 = 2.25$$
$$F = 0.45$$

$$F \times 7 = 0.9 \times 2.5$$
$$F \times 7 = 2.25$$
$$F = 0.32$$

Scale: 1 cm = 0.5 pound

Fig. 3-12:

$$F \times FA = R \times RA$$
$$F \times 1.5 = 4(0.5) \times 5$$
$$F1.5 = 10$$
$$F = 6.67$$

$$F \times 3.75 = 4(0.5) \times 5$$
$$F3.75 = 10$$
$$F = 2.67$$

$$F \times 5.75 = 4(0.5) \times 5$$
$$F5.75 = 10$$
$$F = 1.74$$

Scale: 1 cm = 1 pound

Fig. 3-14: $\text{Sine} = \dfrac{\text{Opposite side}}{\text{Hypotenuse}} = \dfrac{O}{H}$ $\text{Cosine} = \dfrac{\text{Adjacent side}}{\text{Hypotenuse}} = \dfrac{A}{H}$

30°	$0.5 = \frac{O}{8}$	$0.866 = \frac{A}{8}$
	$4.0 = O$	$6.928 = A$
45°	$0.707 = \frac{O}{8}$	$0.707 = \frac{A}{8}$
	$5.656 = O$	$5.656 = A$
60°	$0.866 = \frac{O}{8}$	$0.5 = \frac{A}{8}$
	$6.928 = O$	$4.0 = A$
90°	$1 = \frac{O}{8}$	$0.0 = \frac{A}{8}$
	$8 = O$	$0.0 = A$
120°	*See* 60°	
135°	*See* 45°	
150°	*See* 30°	

Fig. 3-17: $\text{Sine} = \dfrac{\text{Opposite side}}{\text{Hypotenuse}} = \dfrac{O}{H}$ $\qquad$ $\text{Cosine} = \dfrac{\text{Adjacent side}}{\text{Hypotenuse}} = \dfrac{A}{H}$

$30°$ $\qquad$ $0.3420 = \dfrac{O}{4}$ $\qquad\qquad$ $0.9848 = \dfrac{A}{4}$

$\qquad\qquad$ $1.37 = O$ $\qquad\qquad\qquad$ $3.9392 = A$

$45°$ $\qquad$ $0.4226 = \dfrac{O}{4}$ $\qquad\qquad$ $0.9063 = \dfrac{A}{4}$

$\qquad\qquad$ $1.69 = O$ $\qquad\qquad\qquad$ $3.63 = A$

$60°$ $\qquad$ $0.5446 = \dfrac{O}{4}$ $\qquad\qquad$ $0.8387 = \dfrac{A}{4}$

$\qquad\qquad$ $2.18 = O$ $\qquad\qquad\qquad$ $3.35 = A$

Fig. 3-18: $\text{Torque} = \text{Force} \times \text{length}$
$T = 8 \times 1$
$T = 8 \text{ inch-ounces}$

$T = 8 \times 2.25$
$T = 18 \text{ inch-ounces}$

Fig. 3-24, A: $F \times FA = R \times RA$
$F \times 9 = 0.9 \times 3$
$F9 = 2.7$
$F = 0.3$
$0.3 + 0.9 = 1.2$

Fig. 3-24, B: $F \times 3.5 = 0.9 \times 3$
$F3.5 = 2.7$
$F = 0.77$
$0.77 + 0.9 = 1.67$

Fig. 3-24, C: 6.67 from Fig. 3-12
$2 + 6.67 = 8.67$

Fig. 3-24, D: 1.74 from Fig. 3-12
$2 + 1.74 = 3.74$

Scale: 1 cm = 1 pound

APPENDIX B

Equipment and materials

EQUIPMENT AND SOURCES*

Equipment	Source
Supplies	
Ace bandage	Local pharmacy or surgical supply house (e.g., Abbey Medical)
Acetone (solvent for ethyl cyanoacrylate glue)	Local pharmacy or surgical supply house
Cabinets (storage)	Local hardware store
Chair with adjustable seat height for patient	Local pharmacy or surgical supply house
D rings	Fred Sammons, Inc., Box 32, Brookfield, Ill. 60513, or local Tandy Leather Co.
Dressings (e.g., sterile Kling or 4- × 4-inch surgical pads)	Local pharmacy or surgical supply house
Ethyl cyanoacrylate (Permabond)	Local pharmacy or surgical supply house
Finger cuffs	Fred Sammons, Inc.
Fingernail clips (No. 2 dress hooks and eyes)	Local fabric store
Goniometer	Fred Sammons, Inc., or local pharmacy or surgical supply house
Patterns (e.g., paper towels or surgical gloves)	
Pen (not water soluble)	
Petroleum jelly (Vaseline)	Local pharmacy or surgical supply house
Piano wire	Local music company
Rivets (rapid, pop)	Fred Sammons, Inc., or local Tandy Leather Co.
Rubber bands (2 inches wide, No. 30 or 32)†	Fred Sammons, Inc.
Stockinette	Local pharmacy or surgical supply house
Surgical gloves	Local pharmacy or surgical supply house
Tape (adhesive, Micropore)	Local pharmacy or surgical supply house

*Results of a hand splinting questionnaire given to members of the American Society of Hand Therapists, February, 1978.

†Percentages and types of traction used included 48% rubber band, 3% piano wire, and 48% both rubber band and piano wire, in addition to rubber tubing, nylon cord, elastic and banding material.

286

Equipment	Source
Velcro (1-inch hook, plain and adhesive backed; 2-, 1-, and ¾-inch loop)	Fred Sammons, Inc., or local pharmacy or surgical supply house
Tools	
Band saw	Local hardware store
Electric drill and bits	Local hardware store
Files	Local hardware store
Goggles (safety)	Local hardware store
Hammer	Local hardware store
Heat gun and spot heater*	Fred Sammons, Inc., or WFR Corp., 68 Birch St., Ramsey, N.J. 07446
Hydrocollator*	J.A. Preston Corp., 71 Fifth Ave., New York, N.Y. 10003
Jig to construct springs	Local welding shop
Pan (jumbo electric frying – one for dry heat and one for wet heat)*	Fred Sammons, Inc., or local hardware store
Pliers (needlenose)	Local hardware store
Punch (drive and rotary)	Local Tandy Leather Co.
Ruler	Local hardware store
Sander (electric)	Local hardware store
Sandpaper	Local hardware store
Scissors	Local fabric store
Screwdrivers (Phillips and regular)	Local hardware store
Sewing machine	Local fabric store
Sink	
Vise	Local hardware store
Wire cutters	Local hardware store
Wrench (adjustable)	Local hardware store
Splint materials†	
Aquaplast	WFR Corp.
Elastomer and catalyst	Dow Corning Medical Products, Midland, Mich. 48640
Kydex	Rohm & Haas, Independence Mall West, Philadelphia, Pa. 19105
Orthoplast	Johnson & Johnson local distributers, New Brunswick, N.J.
Plaster	Johnson & Johnson
Polycushion	Rohm & Haas
Polyform, Polyfoam	Roylan Medical Products, 14635 Commerce Dr., P.O. Box 555, Menomonee Falls, Wis. 53051
Reston	Fred Sammons, Inc.
Velfoam	Fred Sammons, Inc.
Vinyl	Local Union Carbide plastic supply

*Percentages and types of heat used were 10% wet and 90% both wet and dry.
†Percentages and types of materials used were 74% Aquaplast, 68% plaster, 74% Orthoplast, and 90% Polyform.

EQUIPMENT AND SOURCES – cont'd

Equipment	Source
Commercial splints*	
Capner	Fred Sammons, Inc.
Joint jack	Joint Jack Co., 198 Millstone Rd., Glastonbury, Conn. 06033
LMB Wire-foam	LMB Hand Rehabilitation Products, Inc., 4606 East Alondra Blvd., Dept. 0, Compton, Calif. 90221
Safety pin	J. A. Preston Corp.
Stack	Link America, Inc., 10 Great Meadow Ln., East Hanover, N.J. 07936
Velcro trapper	Local surgical supply house
Web strap	Joint Jack Co.

*Percentages and types of commercial splints used routinely were 23% Capner, 39% joint jack, 42% safety pin, and 23% stack.

MATERIAL ANALYSIS

A. No external heat
  1. Plaster of Paris bandage
    a. Chemical composition and structure formula: Plaster of Paris is manufactured from a solid crystalline material known as gypsum or calcium sulfate. Gypsum is pulverized to break up the crystals and then subjected to intense heat to drive off most of the inherent water of crystallization. The resulting powder is plaster of Paris:

$$2CaSO_4 \cdot 2 H_2O \rightarrow (CaSO_4)_2 \cdot H_2O + 3H_2O$$

    b. Working temperature: 70° to 75° F (21° to 24° C) water.
    c. Physical properties: The setting time is 5 to 8 minutes for fast-setting plaster and 2 to 4 minutes for extrafast-setting plaster. The material is porous and creamy and has serrated edges.
    d. Advantages and disadvantages: Plaster of paris has a low pH loss, is durable, and is inexpensive.
    e. Precautions: Overwrapping the freshly applied cast with an elastic bandage, placing it on a pillow or mattress, covering it with a blanket, or otherwise insulating the cast from free access to the air causes a sharp rise in temperature. Conversely, the most effective way to reduce the temperature of a cast is to increase circulation of air by such means as blowing air over the cast with a circulating fan.
    f. Clinical dermatologic problems: None.
B. Low temperature
  1. Aquaplast
    a. Chemical composition and structure formula: Aquaplast is poly

(epsilon) caprolactone with a small amount of stabilizers and modifiers added. This is a thermoplastic crystalline polyester:

$$(O—O—)_n$$
$$CH_2CH_2CH_2CH_2CH_2\ C$$

b. Working temperature: Softens at 140° F (60° C).

c. Physical properties: Translucent when hard, transparent when soft. Extremely pliable (regular) and more firm (green stripe) versions are available in both $\frac{1}{8}$ and $\frac{1}{16}$-inch thicknesses. Softened Aquaplast clings to dry surfaces and readily self-bonds.

d. Advantages and disadvantages: Aquaplast forms a precise impression of the patient's contours by clinging to the skin as it hardens. Transparency while soft allows observation of the limb through the material as the splint is molded so that potential pressure points can be accurately located, and corrections made. Splints are not affected by body heat or bathing temperatures and are easily cleaned with soap and water. Aquaplast has different molding properties from other low-temperature plastics and requires some practice to use effectively, particularly the most pliable regular material. It is not well suited where dry heat alone is used, which makes Aquaplast excessively sticky. (Recently improved material is less sticky than original.)

e. Precautions: When splinting over fragile skin, open wounds, or stitches, coat the softened Aquaplast with lubricating or petroleum jelly to eliminate the stickiness. Allow extra room when encircling joints because Aquaplast shrinks 2% in both directions as it cools.

f. Clinical dermatologic problems: Occasional skin rash.

2. Orthoplast

a. Chemical composition: Transpolyisoprene.

b. Working temperature: 60° F (15.5° C).

c. Physical properties: This thermoplastic sets within 8 to 10 minutes and is available in plain or perforated sheets.

d. Advantages and disadvantages: Orthoplast is strong, lightweight, washable; has unlimited design possibilities and optimum malleability; adheres to itself without glue or adhesive; is easily united, strapped, or reinforced; and can be reheated and remolded. Color can be changed with nonlead spray paint or epoxy compound.

Precautions: Orthoplast should be stored in the original container away from light and air. Adhesive properties will temporarily deteriorate but may be restored by cleaning the surfaces with nonflammable household spot remover.

e. Clinical dermatologic problems: Occasional skin rash.

3. Polyform

a. Chemical composition and structure formula: Plastic polymer.

    b. Working temperature: 150° to 165° F (65.5° to 74° C) water in 30 to 60 seconds.

    c. Physical properties: Polyform hardens in 3 to 5 minutes, self-bonds, is strong when cooled, and is available in plain or perforated sheets.

    d. Advantages and disadvantages: Polyform is easily molded on the patient; contours precisely to the skin; sets up to be rigid; is reheatable, gas autoclavable, nontoxic, and easy to clean; and involves neither oxone degradation nor shrinking. Polyform will start to soften at 140° F (60° C); therefore, do not leave the splint in a car on a hot day.

    e. Clinical dermatologic problems: No known allergenic reactions.

C. Moderate to high temperature

  1. Kydex

    a. Chemical composition and structure formula: Co-polymer of polyvinyl chloride and acrylic.

    b. Working temperature: 350° F (177° C).

    c. Physical properties: Sheets of Kydex are smooth on one side and textured on the other. The material can be cut with a band saw and finished with a file and sandpaper. Kydex is thermoplastic and rigid.

    d. Advantages and disadvantages: Due to its strength, 3/16 inch Kydex is suitable for outriggers. Kydex cannot be formed on the skin because of the high working temperature and should be fitted on a mold or over a stockinette. If overheated, it will form bubbles and discolor.

    e. Clinical dermatologic problems: Occasional skin rash.

  2. Vinyl

    a. Chemical composition and structure formula: Polyvinyl chloride.

    b. Working temperature: 200° to 225° F (93° to 107° C) in oven or hot water.

    c. Physical properties: Vinyl is a smooth, transparent, blue-tinted sheet. In hot water the material becomes cloudy.

    d. Advantages and disadvantages: Vinyl is slightly elastic when hot, can be cut with a band saw with edges finished by sanding, and has high-impact strength. Vinyl cannot be formed directly on the patient without protective stockinette.

    e. Clinical dermatologic problems: Occasional skin rash.

Forms

SPLINTING AND HAND THERAPY REFERRAL

Name: _____

Address: _____

Phone number: _____

Diagnosis:

Referral for extremity: ☐Right   ☐Left

   ☐ Evaluation and report
   ☐ Evaluation and treatment
      ☐ Range of motion
      ☐ Strengthening
      ☐ Dexterity
      ☐ Sensory reeducation
      ☐ Desensitization
      ☐ Activities of daily living
      ☐ Work/home evaluation
      ☐ Joint protection (arthritic program)
      ☐ Upper extremity prosthetic training
      ☐ Upper extremity Jobst garment measurement and fitting
      ☐ Transcutaneous stimulation
      ☐ Upper extremity Jobst pump
      ☐ Other (specify): _____
   ☐ Splint fabrication:

Continued.

SPLINTING AND HAND THERAPY REFERRAL — cont'd

Check joints desired to be incorporated in splint*:

Immobilize (specify position of joint in degrees)												
						Elbow				Mobilize		
						Ext						
						Flex						
						Wrist						
						Ext						
						Flex						
						UD						
						RD						
					TH		TH					
						CMC						
						Ext						
						Flex						
						Abd						
Ind	Long	Ring	Sm	Th			Th	Ind	Long	Ring	Sm	
						MP						
						Ext						
						Flex						
						RD						
						UD						
						PIP (IP)						
						Ext						
						Flex						
						DIP						
						Ext						
						Flex						

*Ext, Extension; Flex, flexion; RD, radial deviation; UD, ulnar deviation; MP, metacarpophalangeal; PIP, proximal interphalangeal; DIP, distal interphalangeal; ABD, abduction; Th, thumb; Ind, index; Sm, small.

SPLINTING AND HAND THERAPY REFERRAL—cont'd

Describe the function you would like the splint or splints to provide:

The correct fabrication of the splint is important. Therefore, please call for any specific instructions (phone number _____).

INSTRUCTIONS FOR PROPER CARE AND WEARING OF SPLINTS

Your splint was constructed for you; if you have any questions concerning its proper application, fit, or wearing schedule, please contact the hand rehabilitation center.

Please read the following instructions for proper care and wearing of your splint.

Precautions

1. Contact the hand rehabilitation center if your splint causes:
   a. Excessive swelling or stiffness
   b. Severe pain
   c. Pressure area (an irritated skin area resembling the beginning of a blister).
   d. A skin rash or areas in direct contact with the splint.
2. Splints should not be used while operating machinery unless you have specific permission from your physician.
3. Your splint will lose its shape if exposed to heat sources such as radiator, stove, or being left on a car seat during the summer.

Adjustments in rubber band tension

1. A light steady pull (approximately 8 ounces) on your fingers is better than a strong pull.
2. Rubber band tension may be increased if needed by tying knot(s) in the bands. If rubber bands become stretched, replace them with new ones.

Continued.

INSTRUCTIONS FOR PROPER CARE AND WEARING
OF SPLINTS — cont'd

Cleaning your splint

1. Your splint may be cleaned with soap and lukewarm (never hot) water when perspiration and dirt collect inside. To thoroughly clean straps, it may be necessary to scrub them with a small brush.
2. For ink or spots that are difficult to remove, use a cleanser with chlorine.
3. If your sutures have been removed and your wound closed and you have no pins protruding from your skin, you may use talcum powder or corn starch on your hand and arm to help absorb excess moisture.

Wear

☐ Night and rest periods only.
☐ Daytime: for ＿＿ minutes/hours at a time, ＿＿ times a day.
☐ Remove splint every ＿＿＿＿＿＿＿, and do active and/or passive range-of-motion exercises.
☐ ＿＿＿＿＿＿＿＿＿＿＿＿＿＿＿＿＿＿＿＿＿＿＿＿＿

＿＿＿＿＿＿＿＿＿＿＿＿＿＿＿＿＿＿＿＿＿＿＿＿＿

＿＿＿＿＿＿＿＿＿＿＿＿＿＿＿＿＿＿＿＿＿＿＿＿＿

＿＿＿＿＿＿＿＿＿＿＿＿＿＿＿＿＿＿＿＿＿＿＿＿＿

SPLINT CHECKOUT FORM

	Yes	No	Comments
DESIGN			
Does the splint meet general design concepts, including adaptation for:			
1. Individual patient factors			
2. Total utilization time			
3. Simplicity			
4. Optimum function			
5. Optimum sensation			
6. Efficient construction and fit			
7. Ease of application and removal			
8. Exercise regimen			
Does the splint meet specific design concepts, including adaptation for:			
9. Influencing key joints			
10. Attaining purpose			
a. Augment passive motion			
b. Substitute for active motion			
11. Types of forces used			
12. Surface of application			
13. Anatomic variables			
14. Material properties			
MECHANICS			
Does the splint meet specific mechanical concepts, including adaptation for:			
1. Reduction of pressure			
2. Increased mechanical advantage (Ratio of FA to RA)			
3. Optimum rotational force (90°)			
4. Torque			
5. Variance of passive mobility of successive joints			
6. Optimum utilization of parallel forces			
7. Material strength			
8. Elimination of friction			

SPLINT CHECKOUT FORM — cont'd

	Yes	No	Comments
CONSTRUCTION			
Has the splint been fabricated appropriately to provide:			
1. Good cosmesis			
2. Rounded corners			
3. Smooth edges and surfaces			
4. Stable joints			
5. Finished rivets			
6. Ventilation			
7. Secure padding			
8. Secure straps			
FIT			
Has the splint been fitted appropriately to adapt to:			
1. Bony prominences			
2. Dual obliquity			
3. Ligamentous stress			
4. Arches			
5. Joint axis alignment			
6. Skin creases			
7. Kinematic changes			
8. Kinetic concepts			

APPENDIX D

Splint room organization

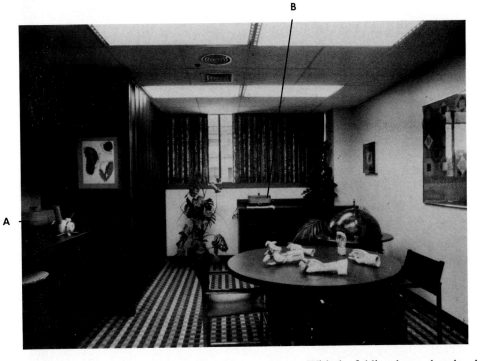

Fig. D-1. This room was designed to serve two purposes. With the folding doors closed and equipment in cabinets, it is used as a small conference room. During patient office hours, it is quickly converted to an efficient splinting area large enough to accommodate two therapists and four or five patients at a time. A "dry" *(A)* and a "wet" *(B)* skillet allow low-temperature splinting materials to be preheated and held at the malleable stage until needed.

A   B

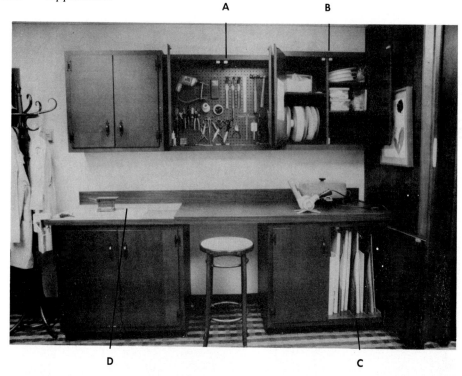

D   C

Fig. D-2. Cabinets are specifically designed for storage of *(A)* tools, *(B)* Velcro, and *(C)* plastics. The finished cabinet top *(D)* slides off to expose a workbench suitable for working with equipment such as hand tools and vises.

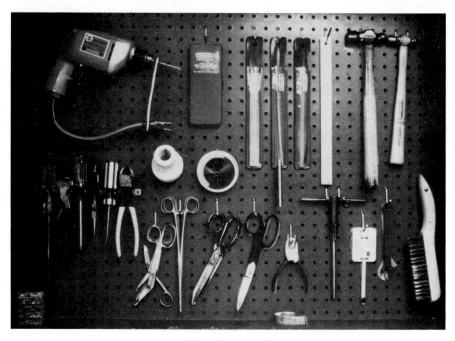

Fig. D-3. Pegboard facilitates efficient storage of small hand tools.

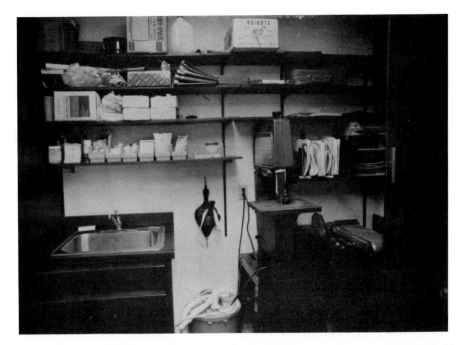

Fig. D-4. Heavy power equipment, a sink, and additional storage shelves are hidden behind the folding door, which may be opened at either end. The sander and band saw are attached to a portable vacuum system to reduce shavings and dust in the area.

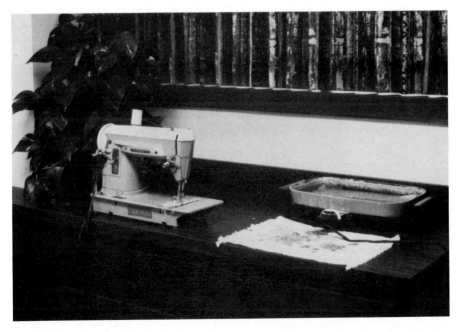

Fig. D-5. A sewing machine facilitates construction of splint components made of Velcro or cloth. A drying towel is placed next to the wet-heat skillet.

APPENDIX E

American Society for Surgery of the Hand clinical assessment recommendations*

A. Sensibility

Apply two-point discrimination with a blunt instrument in a longitudinal axis of the digit. Do not blanch the skin.

Ratings:

1. Normal, less than 6 mm
2. Fair, 6 to 10 mm
3. Poor, 11 to 15 mm
4. Protective, one point perceived
5. Anesthetic, no point perceived

B. Strength

1. Grip: Use a grip dynamometer with the handle preferably in second position. Alteration from this would be recorded as such. Make three successive determinations, record, and calculate percentage relative to pretreatment value as well as to value from contralateral hand.
2. Pinch: Use a standard, commercially available pinch meter. Key pinch is the thumb tip to the radial aspect of the middle phalanx of the index finger and is the most universal and preferred value. Record three successive efforts, and calculate percentage relative to pretreatment as well as to contralateral hand values. (Tip pinch value will be slightly less than key pinch.)
3. Reverse key pinch: Index tip to ulnar tip of thumb. Recordings are the same as those for key pinch.

C. Motion

1. Total passive motion (TPM): Sum of angles formed by MP, PIP, and DIP joints in maximum passive flexion minus the sum of angles of deficit from complete extension at each of these three joints: (MP + PIP + DIP) − (MP + PIP + DIP) = Total flexion − Total extensor lag = TPM.
2. Total active motion (TAM): Sum of angles formed by MP, PIP, and DIP joints in maximum active flexion, that is, fist position, minus total extension

---

*From The hand examination and diagnosis. © 1978 by The American Society for Surgery of the Hand, Aurora, Colo. 80232.

300

deficit at the MP, PIP, and DIP joints with active finger extension. Significant hyperextension at any joint, particularly the PIP and DIP joints, is recorded as a deficit in extension and is included in the total extension deficit. Hyperextension must be considered an abnormal value in swan neck (PIP) and boutonniere deformities (DIP). Comparison of pretreatment and posttreatment TAM values will be significant; however, comparison as a percentage of normal value is invalid. TAM is a term applied to one finger and is:

a. Sum of active MP flexion plus active PIP flexion plus active DIP flexion

b. Minus sum of incomplete active extension if any is present
   (Figs. E-1 to E-3)

D. Vascular status
   Patients who have vascular repair are evaluated in the following manner:
   1. Examination for tissue survival.
   2. Objective evidence of patent vessels by Allen test and/or ultrasonic pulse detector.
   3. Revascularized part examination in resting and postexercise state by one of several methods:
      a. Presence of capillary filling
      b. Physiologic testing such as ultrasonic pulse detector
      When possible, comparison with evaluation before and after 3-minute tourniquet ischemia.

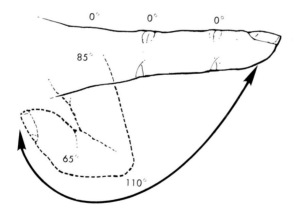

Fig. E-1. Normal range of motion.

Active	Flexion	Extension lack
MP	85°	0°
PIP	110°	0°
DIP	65°	0°
TOTALS	260°	0°

$$\text{TAM} = 260° - 0° = 260°$$

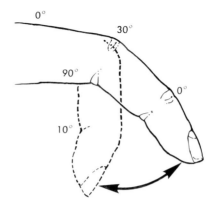

Fig. E-2. Stiff metacarpophalangeal and limited proximal interphalangeal joint extension.

Active	Flexion	Extension lack
MP	0°	0°
PIP	90°	30°
DIP	10°	0°
TOTALS	100°	30°

$$\text{TAM} = 100° - 30° = 70°$$

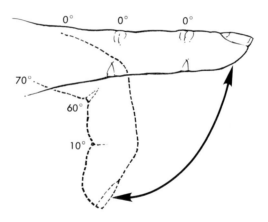

Fig. E-3. Limited metacarpophalangeal and proximal interphalangeal joint flexion with good extension.

Active	Flexion	Extension lack
MP	70°	0°
PIP	60°	0°
DIP	10°	0°
TOTALS	140°	0°

$$\text{TAM} = 140° - 0° = 140°$$

4. Evaluation regarding cold tolerance of the part.
   Ratings:
   a. Failure, no survival
   b. Poor, tissue survival
   c. Fair, objective evidence of patent vessels
   d. Good, function not limited by circulation
   e. Excellent, no cold intolerance

Bibliography

Abouna, J. M.: Splint for mallet finger, Nurs. Mirror PVII, 1966.

American Academy of Orthopaedic Surgeons: Atlas of orthotics: biomechanical principles and application, St. Louis, 1975, The C. V. Mosby Co.

American Academy of Orthopaedic Surgeons: Symposium on Tendon Surgery in the Hand, St. Louis, 1975, The C. V. Mosby Co.

American Academy of Orthopaedic Surgeons: Instructional Lecture Course Series, vol. 27, St. Louis, 1978, The C. V. Mosby Co.

American Society for Surgery of the Hand: Examination and diagnosis, Aurora, Colo., 1978, The Society.

Anderson, M. N.: Upper extremities orthotics, Springfield, Ill., 1965, Charles C Thomas, Publisher.

Ansell, B. M., Williams, J. G., Cheshire, L., Lawton, S., and Haines, R. E.: Farnham Park modular splint system, Rheumatol. Phys. Med. 11:334-336, 1972.

Araicoj, J. L., and Ortiz, J. M.: An internal wire splint for adduction contracture of the thumb, Plast. Reconstr. Surg. 48:339-342, 1971.

Barr, N.: Peripheral nerve lesions of the upper limb and lively splints, Physiotherapy 57:533-538, 1971.

Barr, N.: The hand: principles and techniques of simple splintmaking in rehabilitation, London, 1975, Butterworth & Co. (Publishers), Ltd.

Basmajian, J. V.: Practical functional anatomy. In Hunter, J. M., Schneider, L. H., Mackin, E. J., and Bell, J. A., editors: Rehabilitation of the hand, St. Louis, 1978, The C. V. Mosby Co.

Beasley, R. W.: The addition of dynamic splinting to hand casts, Plast. Reconstr. Surg. 44:507, 1969.

Becker, C. G.: Adaption of Bunnell block, Am. J. Occup. Ther. 29:108, 1975.

Bennett, R. L.: Orthotic devices to prevent deformities of the hand in rheumatoid arthritis, Arthritis Rheum. 8:1006-1018, 1965.

Betts, G. A.: An adjustable plastazote splint for the hand or arm, Nurs. Times 66:1556-1557, 1970.

Bloch, R., and Evans, M. G.: An inflatable splint for the spastic hand, Arch. Phys. Med. Rehabil. 58:179-180, 1977.

Blue, A. I., Spira, M., and Hardy, S. B.: Repair of extensor tendon injuries of the hand, Am. J. Surg. 132:128-132, 1976.

Boyes, J. H., editor: Bunnell's surgery of the hand, ed. 4, Philadelphia, 1964, J. B. Lippincott Co.

Boyes, J. H., editor: Bunnell's surgery of the hand, ed. 5, Philadelphia, 1970, J. B. Lippincott Co.

Bradley, K.: Basic splinting manual, Unpublished handout, Indianapolis, 1968, Indiana University Medical Center School of Occupational Therapy.

Bradley, K., Fess, E., and Keal, J.: Basic splinting manual, Unpublished handout, Indianapolis, 1972, Indiana University Medical School of Occupational Therapy.

Brand, P. W.: The reconstruction of the hand in leprosy, Ann. R. Coll. Surg. Engl. 11:350, 1952.

Brand, P. W.: Rehabilitation of the hand in leprosy. In Cramer, L. M., and Chase, R. A., editors: Symposium on the hand, vol. 3, St. Louis, 1971, The C. V. Mosby Co.

Brand, P. W.: Rehabilitation of the hand with motor and sensory impairment, Orthop. Clin. North Am. 4:1135-1139, 1973.

Brand, P. W.: Biomechanics of tendon transfer, Orthop. Clin. North Am. 5:205-230, 1974.

Brown, P. W.: The management of phalangeal and metacarpal fractures, Surg. Clin. North Am. 53:1393-1437, 1973.

Brumstrom, S.: Clinical kinesiology, ed. 3, Philadelphia, 1972, F. A. Davis Co.

Buchan, N. G.: Experience with thermoplastic splints in the post-burn hand, Br. J. Plast. Surg. 28:8193-8197, 1975.

304

Buckner, G.: A dynamic finger splint, Am. J. Occup. Ther. **27:**39, 1973.

Bunch, W., and Keagy, R.: Principles of orthotic treatment, St. Louis, 1976, The C. V. Mosby Co.

Bunnell, S.: Surgery of the hand, Philadelphia, 1944, J. B. Lippincott Co.

Bunnell, S.: Splinting the hand. In American Academy of Orthopaedic Surgeons: Instructional course lectures, vol. IX, Ann Arbor, 1952, J. W. Edwards.

Bunnell, S., and Howard, L.: Additional elastic hand splints, J. Bone Joint Surg. [Am.] **32:**226-228, 1950.

Buntine, J. A., and Holthouse, R. L.: Simple physiotherapy for hand injuries, Med. J. Aust. **2:**187-190, 1970.

Butts, D. E., and Goldberg, M. J.: Congenital absence of the radius: the occupational therapist and a new orthosis, Am. J. Occup. Ther. **31:**95-100, 1977.

Cailliet, R.: Hand pain and impairment, Philadelphia, 1975, F. A. Davis Co.

Capener, N.: Lively splints, Physiotherapy **53:** 371-374, 1967.

Carr, K.: Hand splints for rheumatoid arthritis, Can. J. Occup. Ther. **35:**17-18, 1978.

Charait, S. E.: A comparison of volar and dorsal splinting of the hemiplegic hand, Am. J. Occup. Ther. **22:**319-322, 1968.

Collins, R. D.: Illustrated manual of neurologic diagnosis, Philadelphia, 1962, J. B. Lippincott Co.

Cramer, L. M., and Chase, R. A.: Symposium on the hand, vol. 3, St. Louis, 1971, The C. V. Mosby Co.

Craver, P. N.: Typing splints for the quadriplegic patient, Am. J. Occup. Ther. **29:**551, 1975.

Curtis, R. M.: Fundamental principles of tendon transfer, Orthop. Clin. North Am. **5:**231-242, 1974.

Czap, L.: Orthotic management of the rheumatoid hand, South. Med. J. **59:**1115-1117, 1966.

Daniel, R., and Terzis, J.: Reconstructive microsurgery, Boston, 1977, Little, Brown & Co.

Doyle, J. R., and Blythe, W.: The finger flexor tendon sheath and pulleys: anatomy and reconstruction. In American Academy of Orthopaedic Surgeons: Symposium on Tendon Surgery in the Hand, St. Louis, 1975, The C. V. Mosby Co.

Duran, R. J., Houser, R. G., and Stover, M. G.: Management of flexor tendon lacerations in zone 2 using controlled passive motion postoperatively. In Hunter, J. M., et al., editors: Rehabilitation of the hand, St. Louis, 1978, The C. V. Mosby Co.

Dworecka, F., Wisham, L. H., and Smith, R.: A new device for the restoration of partially amputated hands, Mt. Sinai J. Med. **38:**462-469, 1971.

Eaton, R. G., and Littler, J. W.: Joint injuries and their sequelae, Clin. Plast. Surg. **3:**87-98, 1976.

Eaton, R. G.: Joint injuries of the hand, Springfield, Ill., 1971, Charles C Thomas, Publisher.

Elliott, R. A., Jr.: Splints for mallet and boutonniere deformities, Plast. Reconstr. Surg. **52:** 282-285, 1973.

Engel, W. H., Kmiotek, M. S., Hoht, J. P., French, J., Barnerias, M. J., and Siebens, A. A.: A functional splint for grasp driven by wrist extension, Arch. Phys. Med. Rehabil. **48:** 43-52, 1967.

Evans, E. B.: Orthopaedic measures in the treatment of severe burns, J. Bone Joint Surg. **48A:** 643, 1966.

Fisher, T. R.: The mallet finger and its treatment, Nurs. Mirror IV-VI, 1966.

Flatt, A. E.: The care of the rheumatoid hand, ed. 3, St. Louis, 1974, The C. V. Mosby Co.

Flatt, A. E.: The care of congenital hand anomalies, St. Louis, 1977, The C. V. Mosby Co.

Flatt, A. E.: The care of minor hand injuries, ed. 4, St. Louis, 1979, The C. V. Mosby Co.

Flynn, J. E.: Hand surgery, Baltimore, 1966, The Williams & Wilkins Co.

Gault, S. J., and Spyker, M. J.: Beneficial effect of immobilization of joints in rheumatoid and related arthritides: a splint study using sequential analysis, Arthritis Rheum. **12:**34-44, 1969.

Gibbs, B. L.: Functional splint after flexor pollicis longus repair, Am. J. Occup. Ther. **23:**344-345, 1969.

Goodman, C. R., Delaney, H. F., and Patterson, P. T.: The use of the Prenyl RIC splint in the early rehabilitation of the upper extremity, Am. J. Occup. Ther. **24:**119-121, 1970.

Grahn, E. C.: A power unit for functional hand splints, Bull. Prosthet. Res. **10:**52-56, 1970.

Grant, J. C.: Grant's atlas of anatomy, ed. 6, Baltimore, 1972, The Williams & Wilkins Co.

Gray, H.: Gray's anatomy of the human body, Am. ed. 29, edited by C. M. Goss, Philadelphia, 1973, Lea & Febiger.

Griffin, J. M., and Lissner, G.: Tape splinting for mallet finger, Mo. Med. **69:**813, 1973.

Gruen, H.: A postoperative dynamic splint for the rheumatoid hand, Am. J. Occup. Ther. **24:** 284, 1970.

Haines, R.: The mechanism of rotation of the first carpometacarpal joint, J. Anat. **78:**44, 1944.

Hirsch, G.: Tensile properties during tendon

healing, Copenhagen, 1974, Einar Munksgaard.

Hollinshead, H. W.: Anatomy for surgeons, vol. 3: The back and limbs, New York, 1969, Harper & Row, Publishers.

Hollis, L. I.: Splint substitutes, Am. J. Occup. Ther. **21:**139-145, 1967.

Hoppenfeld, S.: Physical examination of the spine and extremities, New York, 1976, Appleton-Century-Crofts.

Hueston, J. T., and Tubiana, R.: Dupuytren's disease, New York, 1974, Grune & Stratton, Inc.

Hunter, J. M., Schneider, L. H., Mackin, E. J., and Bell, J. A., editors: Rehabilitation of the hand, St. Louis, 1978, The C. V. Mosby Co.

Jensen, A., and Chenoweth, H.: Statics and strengths of materials, New York, 1975, McGraw-Hill Book Co.

Johnson, C. J., and Graham, W. P.: Use of thermoplastic splints in the treatment of burned hands, Plast. Reconstr. Surg. **44:**399-400, 1969.

Johnson, M., and Cohen, M.: The hand atlas, Springfield, Ill., 1975, Charles C Thomas, Publisher.

Jones, R. F., and James, R.: A simple functional hand splint for C5-6 quadriplegia, Med. J. Aust. **1:**988-1000, 1970.

Kapandji, I. A.: The physiology of the joints, vol. I: Upper limb, Edinburgh, 1970, Churchill Livingstone.

Kaplan, E. B.: Functional and surgical anatomy of the hand, ed. 2, Philadelphia, 1965, J. B. Lippincott Co.

Kaplan, E. B.: Anatomy and kinesiology of the hand. In Flynn, J. E., editor: Hand surgeries, ed. 2, Baltimore, 1975, The Williams & Wilkins Co.

Kay, H. W.: Clinical evaluation of the Engen plastic hand orthosis, Artif. Limbs **13:**13-26, 1969.

Kester, N. C., and Lehneis, H. R.: A combined ADL–long opponens orthosis, Arch. Phys. Med. Rehabil. **50:**219-222, 1969.

Kleinert, H., Kutz, J., and Cohen, M.: Primary repair of zone 2 flexor tendon lacerations. In American Academy of Orthopaedic Surgeons: Symposium on tendon surgery in the hand, St. Louis, 1975, The C. V. Mosby Co.

Knapp, M. E.: Orthotics: bracing in upper extremity, Postgrad. Med. **43:**215-219, 1968.

Kolumban, S. L.: The use of dynamic and static splints in straightening contracted proximal interphalangeal joints in leprosy patients: a comparative study. Presented at the Forty-seventh Annual Conference of the American Physical Therapy Association, Washington, D.C., 1960.

Kolumban, S. L.: M. H. thesis. New York, 1967, New York University.

Kolumban, S. L.: The role of static and dynamic splints, physiotherapy techniques and time in straightening contractures of the interphalangeal joints, Lepr. India 323-328, 1969.

Kopell, H. P., and Thompson, W. A. L.: Peripheral entrapment neuropathies, Baltimore, 1963, The Williams & Wilkins Co.

Krusen, F., Kottke, F., and Ellwood, P.: Handbook of physical medicine and rehabilitation, Philadelphia, 1971, W. B. Saunders Co.

Lampe, E. W.: Surgical anatomy of the hand. In Clinical symposia, New York, 1969, Ciba Pharmaceutical Co., Division of Ciba-Geigy Corp.; illustrations by F. H. Netter.

Landsmeer, J.: Atlas of anatomy of the hand, Edinburgh, 1976, Churchill Livingstone.

Laskin, R. S.: Simple splint for finger injuries, Postgrad. Med. **4:**174-175, 1970.

LaVore, J. S., and Marshall, J. H.: Expedient splinting of the burned patient, Phys. Ther. **52:**1036-1042, 1972.

Lesiak, A., and Seyfried, A.: Splinting of the rheumatoid hand in an apparatus in cases of ulnar deviation in the metacarpophalangeal joints, Reumatologia **7:**247-253, 1969.

Levinson, I.: Introduction to mechanics, ed. 2, Englewood Cliffs, N. J., 1968, Prentice-Hall, Inc.

Licht, S. H., and Kamenetz, H. L., editors: Orthotics etcetera, New Haven, Conn., 1966, Elizabeth Licht, Publisher.

Lindsay, W. K.: Hand injuries in children, Clin. Plast. Surg. **3:**65-75, 1976.

Littler, J. W., Cramer, L. M., and Smith, J. W., editors: Symposium on Reconstructive Hand Surgery, St. Louis, 1974, The C. V. Mosby Co.

Malick, M. H.: Manual on static hand splinting, Pittsburgh, 1972, Harmarville Rehabilitation Center.

Malick, M. H.: Manual on dynamic hand splinting with thermoplastic materials, Pittsburgh, 1974, Harmarville Rehabilitation Center.

Malick, M. H.: A preliminary prosthesis for the partially amputated hand, Am. J. Occup. Ther. **29:**479-482, 1975.

Marble, H. C.: The hand, a manual and atlas for the general surgeon, Philadelphia, 1960, W. B. Saunders Co.

Mason, M. L., and Allen, H. S.: The rate of healing of tendons: an experimental study of tensile strength, Ann. Surg. **113:**424-459, 1941.

McCluer, S., and Conry, J. E.: Modifications of

the wrist-driven flexor hinge splint, Arch. Phys. Med. Rehabil. **52**:233-235, 1971.

McDougall, D.: Modern concepts in hand orthotics, Hand **7**:58-62, 1975.

McElfresh, E. C., Dobyns, J. H., and O'Brien, E. T.: Management of fracture-dislocation of the proximal interphalangeal joints by extension-block splinting, J. Bone Joint Surg. [Am.] **54.8**:1705-1711, 1972.

McFarland, S. R., Laenger C. J. S. R., Francis, P. N., and Ziperman, H. H.: Fiber reinforced composites for orthotics, prosthetics, and mobility aids, Biomed. Sci. Instrum. **11**:151-156, 1975.

McFarlane, R. M., and Hampole, M. K.: Treatment of extensor tendon injuries of the hand, Can. J. Surg. **16**:366-375, 1973.

McKenzie, M. W.: The Ratchet handsplint, Am. J. Occup. Ther. **27**:477-479, 1973.

Melvin, J. L.: Rheumatic disease: occupational therapy and rehabilitation, Philadelphia, 1977, F. A. Davis Co.

Merletti, R., Acimovic, R., Grobelnik, S., and Cvilak, G.: Electrophysiological orthosis for the upper extremity in hemiplegia: feasibility study, Arch. Phys. Med. Rehabil. **56**:507-513, 1975.

Michon, J., and Moberg, E., editors: Traumatic nerve lesions of the upper limb, Group d'Etude de la Main Monographs 2, Edinburgh, 1975, Churchill Livingstone.

Michon, J., and Pillet, J.: The GEM dynamic hand splint, Hand **6**:295-296, 1974.

Mikic, Z., and Helal, B.: The treatment of the mallet finger by the Oakley splint, Hand **6**:76-81, 1974.

Milford, L.: Retaining ligaments of the digits of the hand, Philadelphia, 1968, W. B. Saunders Co.

Milford, L.: The hand, St. Louis, 1971, The C. V. Mosby Co.

Millender, L. H., and Philips, C.: Uses of the proximal interphalangeal joint gutter splint, Am. J. Occup. Ther. **27**:8-13, 1973.

Moberg, E.: Dressings, splints and post-operative care in hand surgery, Surg. Clin. North Am. **44**:941, 1964.

Moberg, E.: Surgical treatment for absent single-hand grip and elbow extension in quadriplegia. J. Bone Joint Surg. [Am.] **57**:196, 1975.

Nalebuff, E., and Millender, L.: Robert B. Brigham Hospital dynamic hand splint, Midland, Mich., Dow Corning Medical Products.

Namasivayam, P. R.: A spiral splint for claw fingers, Lepr. India **48**:258-260, 1976.

Napier, J. R.: The form and function of the carpo-metacarpal joint of the thumb, J. Anat. **89**:362-369, 1955.

Napier, J. R.: The prehensile movements of the human hand, J. Bone Joint Surg. [Br.] **38**:902-913, 1956.

Netter, F. H.: Illustrations for Surgical anatomy of the hand. In Clinical symposia, New York, 1969, Ciba-Geigy Corp.

Newmeyer, W. L., and Kilgore, E. S., Jr.: Management of the burned hand, Phys. Ther. **57**:16-23, 1977.

Nicolle, F. V., and Presswell, D.: A valuable splint for the rheumatoid hand, Hand **7**:67-69, 1975.

Niehuss, J. E.: An improved method to attach straps to plaster splints, Phys. Ther. **45**:1059, 1965.

Oakes, T. W., Ward, J. R., Gray, R. M., Klauber, M. R., and Moody, P. M.: Family expectations and arthritis patient compliance to a hand resting splint regimen, J. Chronic Dis. **22**:757-764, 1970.

Overton, J., and Wolcott, L. E.: The role of splints in the prevention of deformity in the rheumatoid hand and wrist, Mo. Med. **63**:423-427, 1966.

Patterson, R. P., Halpern, D., and Kubicek, W. G.: A proportionally controlled externally powered hand splint, Arch. Phys. Med. Rehabil. **52**:434-438, 1971.

Peacock, E., Jr.: Dynamic splinting for the prevention and correction of deformities, J. Bone Joint Surg. [Am.] **34**:789-796, 1952.

Perry, J., Hsu, J., Barber, L., and Holler, M. M.: Orthosis in patients with brachial plexus injuries, Arch. Phys. Med. Rehabil. **55**:134-137, 1974.

Phelps, P. E., and Weeks, P. M.: Management of the thumb-index web space contracture, Am. J. Occup. Ther. **30**:543-550, 1976.

Quest, I. M., and Corderly, J.: A functional ulnar deviation cuff for the rheumatoid deformity, Am. J. Occup. Ther. **25**:32-37, 1971.

Quintner, J. L.: Hand splints in "Prenyl" for rheumatoid arthritis. A preliminary report, Ann. Phys. Med. **9**:280-281, 1968.

Rank, B. K., Wakefield, A. R., and Hueston, J. T.: Surgery of repair as applied to hand injuries, ed. 3, Baltimore, 1968, The Williams & Wilkins Co.

Rasch, P., and Burke, R.: Kinesiology and applied anatomy, ed. 5, Philadelphia, 1974, Lea & Febiger.

Reardon, J. C.: Occupational therapy treatment of the patient with thermally injured upper extremity, Major Probl. Clin. Surg. **19**:127-147, 1976.

Ries, D. A.: A new material for splinting in hand surgery, Mo. Med. **64**:843, 1967.

Rizzo, F., Hamilton, B. B., and Keagy, R. D.: Orthotics research evaluation framework, Arch. Phys. Med. Rehabil. **56:**304-308, 1975.

Rockwood, C., and Green, D.: Fractures, vols. 1 and 2, Philadelphia, 1975, J. B. Lippincott Co.

Ruch, C., and Dommisse, G. F.: A myo-electric hand splint for quadriplegia, S. Afr. J. Surg. **5:** 97-103, 1967.

Rusk, H. A.: Rehabilitation medicine, ed. 4, St. Louis, 1977, The C. V. Mosby Co.

Saferin, E. H., and Posch, I. L.: Secretan's disease: post-traumatic hard edema of the dorsum of the hand, Plast. Reconstr. Surg. **58:**703-707, 1976.

Salisbury, R. E., and Palm, L.: Dynamic splinting for dorsal burns of the hand, Plast. Reconstr. Surg. **51:**226-228, 1973.

Seddon, H.: Surgical disorders of the peripheral nerves, Baltimore, 1972, The Williams & Wilkins Co.

Silverstein, F., French, J., and Siebens, A.: A myoelectric hand splint, Am. J. Occup. Ther. **28:**99-101, 1974.

Simard, T. G., and Ladd, H. W.: Hand orthotic device influence on fine neuromuscular control, Arch. Phys. Med. Rehabil. **57:**258-263, 1976.

Skoog, T.: Plastic surgery: new methods and refinements, Stockholm, 1974, Almqvist & Wilksell.

Snow, R. S.: Constructing an improved splint for mallet finger deformity, Plast. Reconstr. Surg. **52:**586-588, 1973.

Souter, W. A.: Splintage in the rheumatoid hand, Hand **3:**144-151, 1971.

Spelbring, L. M.: Splinting the arthritic hand, Am. J. Occup. Ther. **20:**40-41, 1966.

Staden, D. V.: An approach to the extensively injured hand, S. Afr. Med. J. **47:**380-381, 1973.

Strickland, J. W., et al.: Factors influencing digital performance following phalangeal fractures. Presented at American Society for Surgery of the Hand, Annual Symposium, 1979, San Francisco.

Sunderland, S.: Nerves and nerve injuries, Baltimore, 1968, The Williams & Wilkins Co.

Sutcliffe, B., and Clark, C.: A polythene and plastazote hand-resting splint, Physiotherapy **58:**138-139, 1972.

Swanson, A. B.: Flexible implant resection arthroplasty in the hand and extremities, St. Louis, 1973, The C. V. Mosby Co.

Swanson, A. B., and Coleman, J. D.: Corrective bracing needs of the rheumatoid arthritic wrist, Am. J. Occup. Ther. **20:**38, 1966.

Taleisnik, J.: Wrist anatomy, function and injury. In American Academy of Orthopaedic sur-geons: Instructional Lecture Course Series, vol. 27, St. Louis, 1978, The C. V. Mosby Co.

Thompson, L., Gosling, C., and Hayes, E.: A facial moulage technique for the plastic surgeon. Presented at the Annual Meeting of the American Society of Plastic and Reconstructive Surgeons, October 5, 1971, Montreal.

Torres, J.: Little finger splint, Am. J. Occup. Ther. **29:**230, 1965.

Truong, X. T.: Fluidic power and control for hand orthosis and prosthesis, Arch. Phys. Med. Rehabil. **54:**91-96, 1973.

Truong, X. T., White, C. F., and Canterbury, R. A.: Modification of flexor tenodesis splint, Arch. Phys. Med. Rehabil. **50:**97–99, 1969.

Tupper, J. W.: A compression arthrodesis device for small joints of the hands, Hand **4:**62-64, 1972.

Vanbrocklin, J. D.: Splinting the rheumatoid hand, Arch. Phys. Med. Rehabil. **47:**262-265, 1966.

Varian, J. P.: The ridged plaster volar slab, Hand **7:**78-80, 1975.

Von Lanz, T., and Wachsmuth, W.: Praktische anatomie, 1959. In Boyes, J. H., editor: Bunnell's surgery of the hand, ed. 5, Philadelphia, 1970, J. B. Lippincott Co.

Von Prince, K. M. P., and Yeakel, M. H.: The splinting of burn patients, Springfield, 1974, Charles C Thomas, Publisher.

Von Prince, K. M. P., Curren, P. W., and Pruitt, B. H., Jr.: Application of fingernail hooks in splinting of burned hands, Am. J. Occup. Ther. **24:**556-559, 1970.

Wadsworth, T. G.: The traction hand splint, Hand **5:**268-269, 1973.

Watson-Jones, R.: Fractures and joint injuries, vol. 1, ed. 4, Baltimore, 1952, The Williams & Wilkins Co.

Waylett, J., and Barbern, L.: Upper extremity bracing of the severely athetoid mental retardate, Am. J. Occup. Ther. **25:**402-407, 1971.

Weckesser, E.: Treatment of hand injuries—preservation and restoration of function, Chicago, 1974, Yearbook Medical Publishers, Inc. (The Press of Case Western Reverse University, Ltd.).

Weeks, P. M., and Wray, R. C.: Management of acute hand injuries: biological approach, ed. 2, St. Louis, 1973, The C. V. Mosby Co.

Williams, J. G.: Splints for the rheumatoid hand, Br. Med. J. **1:**106, 1970.

Williams, M., and Lissner, H.: Biomechanics of human motions, Philadelphia, 1962, W. B. Saunders Co.

Wolcott, L. E.: Orthotic management of the spastic hand, South. Med. J. **59:**971-974, 1966.

Wood, H. L.: Prevention of deformity in the insensitive hand: the role of the therapist, Am. J. Occup. Ther. **23:**487-560, 1969.

Wynn Parry, C. B.: Management of the stiff joint, Hand **3:**169-171, 1971.

Wynn Parry, C. B., et al.: Rehabilitation of the hand, ed. 3, London, 1973, Butterworth & Co. (Publishers), Ltd.

Wynn Parry, C. B.: Restoration of hand function rehabilitation of the injured hand, Trans. Med. Soc. Lond. **90:**101-104, 1974.

Wynn Parry, C. B., Harper, D., Fletcher, I., Dean, P. E., Knight, P. N., and Robinson, P. R.: New types of lively splints for peripheral nerve lesions affecting the hand, Hand **2:**31-38, 1970.

Yeakel, M. H.: Polypropylene hinges for hand splints, J. Bone Joint Surg. [Am.] **48:**955-956, 1966.

Zancolli, E.: Structural and dynamic bases of hand surgery, Philadelphia, 1968, J. B. Lippincott Co.

Zoeckler, A. A., and Nicholas, J. J.: Prenyl hand splint for rheumatoid arthritis, Phys. Ther. **49:** 377-379, 1969.

Zrubecky, G., and Stoger, M.: The orthosis for restoration of prehensile function in tetraplegics, Paraplegia **11:**228-237, 1973.

Index

310